100 DROPS OF WATER

practical steps for filling your soul when you feel empty

HELEN JOY GEORGE

Copyright © 2025 by Helen Joy George

Cover art by Whitney Anderson

All rights reserved.

No part of this book may be reproduced in any form or by any electronic or mechanical means, including information storage and retrieval systems, without written permission from the author, except for the use of brief quotations in a book review.

Dedicated to Sullivan, my boy full of wonder, who reminds me that the simplest things are the best things.

How to read this book

This book is not meant to be read straight through like a novel. It is meant to be savored and searched, leafed through and guided to the right pages. I am hoping that it feels like a worn out captain's log that has all the coordinates of a good journey etched into its pages.

This is also a guide not a "how to." There are so many ways that a person can show up —big or small. Some of these things might feel absolutely life-changing in a way that makes you want to adopt it into your daily life; some things might be a one time experience that you never want to try again.

There are many ways to fill the soul; however the only thing you must do is to take that first small step of action.

How to read this book

This book isn't really meant to be read in the immediate aftermath of tragedy or as a cure for clinical depression that has you bedridden. No dear one, for that you must allow time, rest, medication (at times), and grieving. No, this book is for the *after*, when you find yourself aching to be filled back up again.

Over the years, I have found many ways to come alive, to fill my cup—my soul. And I've written them here…for me and for you. When that feeling comes, we can flip open this book and choose something to do, an action step to take. It may only be a drop in an empty cup, but if we keep showing up for ourselves, suddenly, those drops will turn into fullness.

A little about me

I feel empty a lot. I have since some of my earliest memories were formed. I think it's a combination of trauma, inherited brain chemicals, and the state of our modern society. Regardless, this highly sensitive person who would often be accused of being melancholy, knows quite a lot about feeling empty.

I've been in therapy for decades and take medication every day for Bipolar I Disorder. I am constantly striving to come into a place of wholeness—which I have been feeling much more than I used to. But, despite my fight for wellness, I still experience moments, days, and sometimes seasons of emptiness. Regardless of what we call it (depression, apathy, overstimulation, should I move to Europe), I find myself feeling stuck there, waving blindly in the dark

A little about me

to grab hold of something to pull me back. Over the many dark seasons of my soul, I have collected little practical ways that I can take to feel better. I've had to write them down because in darkness I can never quite remember what they are.

Maybe you know exactly how that feels.

I know that regardless of why, more people than we think experience days, weeks, or seasons of feeling stuck, empty, and depressed. It's just part of being human. Unfortunately, in this modern life, this life that is often disconnected from community, nature, and simple slow pleasures—it can feel impossible to find your way back to feeling whole. We get on our devices, we get advertised to, we compare our lives with the highlight reel of others, we pass by life's most beautiful and simple gifts; gifts that are guaranteed to fill our souls.

I started writing this book the month I left my 17-year marriage that had left me a shell of a person. I felt irreversibly damaged. When confronted with lots of solo time without my kids, I knew I had a choice. . .I could numb myself in a hundred ways, or I could fight to fill back up, one drop at a time.

It's now been 4 years, I'm blissfully remarried to the love of my life; I have a peaceful home, my children are happy, I get to write books and make art.

I have a beautiful life. And I still find myself needing the words written in this book when I lose my way. I hope my years of trial and error, and the wisdom collected along the way will bring you peace, abundance, presence, connection, and your soul filled to overflowing.

1

Touch grass...or dirt

Maybe you are searching among the branches for what only appears in the roots.
—*Rumi*

When I have nothing left to give, when I feel empty and drained of energy, I crawl myself outside and lay like a starfish on the grass of my front yard, even at the risk of my neighbors seeing me. The sun warms me; I let every inch of my body sink into the earth, I let it hold me, cradling me in a way that soothes me to my core. Within minutes, my racing mind whirs at a slower speed and I feel connected to so much more than myself and my problems. I've been doing this since I was a child, but until recently didn't know that what I called "being a starfish" had a name: grounding.

The healing benefits of grounding are scientifically proven. The energy of the earth can recharge us just by being in contact with it.

You can lay like me, outstretched and open. You can walk barefoot on dirt or grass, you can sit on the walking path next to your work and just…be held. Being (literally) connected to the earth is one of the most transformative and simple ways to fill yourself up again. Renew yourself, take your shoes off and touch some grass!

2

Toast

We'll laugh and toast to nothing, and smash our empty glasses down.

—Joni Mitchel

I have a friend named Elise who has a mural painted on her garage. It's blue with flowers and colors that pop. It reads, "Celebrate everything"

This is not just a cute little phrase that looks good to the neighborhood, this is her mantra in life.

And why shouldn't we be celebrating every chance we get? Why shouldn't we inject joy into our days?

I started doing little toasts when my kids were little and I wanted to mark milestones with a celebration. Maybe it was the start of summer break, the fact that someone made an "a", or simply because we pulled the wedding china out for dinner. I would buy sparkling grape juice and everyone was primed for the celebration.

Toasts to try:

Cheers to Tuesday!

Cheers to making it through another day!

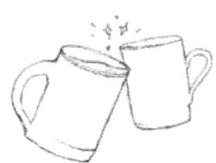

Cheers to friendship!

Cheers to spring!

Cheers to you, middle child who is just killing it at middle school!

Cheers to finishing the laundry for one brief second!

. . .

You can use your grandmother's crystal glasses, paper cups from Christmas 4 years ago…you can toast fancy champagne or capri suns. You can toast with strangers, friends, lovers, or even yourself in the reflection of the kitchen window.

Celebration is contagious, spread it!

3

Stand in a river

No man ever steps in the same river twice, for it's not the same river and he's not the same man.

—Heraclitus

I don't care who you are. I don't care if you are old or young, rich or poor, outdoorsy or a city person, standing in a river will change you. No one comes out of one the same as they went in.

Too many times to count, I have driven to the river, blinded by tears and heavy laden only to have it melt away as I walked into the water. The rivers in the mountains where I live are bitter cold all through the year. Sometimes I can only stand to dip my feet in. Other days, I can't help but plunge into the deep parts and be baptized, suspended in the comfort of the waters.

Something I love about rivers is that they are always moving. I think I go there when I feel stuck because rivers are the opposite of stuck. Even if a branch blocks up a path, a river will find a new way —it's always shifting, changing, and continuing on.

This medicine is simple and free. Go. Find a river near you, or even a shallow creek. Yelp with delight as the cool waters shock you, laugh as you stumble on the rocks, cry and let your tears fall into the water. You are not too much for a river.

4

Print photos

When words become unclear, I shall focus with photographs.
　—*Ansel Adams*

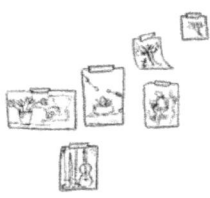

My house is lovely. I have decorated it with years of thrifted treasures; oil paintings, antiques, a bird's nest I found one fall day last year, and carefully framed photos. My home is an extension of my soul. But even with all that thoughtful decor, my favorite part of my home is the photo wall where I have taped cell phone snapshots with off-brand scotch tape in no pattern whatsoever. And without fail, when people first come to my home, that is also where they gravitate to. Yes my Instagram has these same photos saved in a cloud somewhere but having them physically on my wall reminds me of so much goodness.

It's a reminder of the time we played hooky from school and got ice cream cones, the beautiful sunset my daughter twirled under after a particularly harrowing winter, the love, the fun, the special moments that are after all, not the big moments.

I used to carefully print and frame photos every few months, sometimes switching out photos as my children grew. That process became overwhelming and expensive. But I still wanted the ritual of choosing moments to print. That is when I decided to have an imperfect photo wall. And I love it. My children love it and the process of choosing, printing, and viewing is absolutely a meditative experience ripe with presence.

The way I make printing photos enjoyable and not stressful is choosing them from my phone, putting on a good playlist, setting a timer, letting go of any expectations of perfection or "getting all the good shots ordered," and just adding 24-48 (depending on my budget) photos to my Print Studio app. I like a nice blend of candids, detail shots (like my daughter's hands in the river), and selfies. I order them, and then I tape them up with a ceremonious respect.

And it never gets old to remember there's so much good we let pass by, and having a photo in our hands lets us keep it a little bit longer.

5

Go for a walk

Walking is a man's best medicine.
  —Hippocrates

If I were a betting woman, the one drop of water that I would recommend to 100% change how you feel at any given time, I would choose the very simple act of taking a walk. A walk is a mental health Epipen.

Whether it is anxiety, ruminating, or just generally feeling like not wanting to be here anymore, walking will change the way you feel in that moment. It might not last long, and doing it once will certainly not move you out of a season of emptiness, but if you want to feel better. . .take a walk. I have never felt worse after a walk.

It doesn't have to be long. I've taken a day

changing 3 minute walk before. It doesn't have to be fast. You don't have to wear special clothes or shoes, you don't have to walk like anyone else.

Walking is just putting one foot in front of the other. And that motion stimulates the brain with bilateral stimulation. This can reduce racing thoughts, it can calm the nervous system, it can put you in a sort of rhythmic trance in which you can let go of what's ailing you.

Maybe you want to start with 5 minutes. Maybe you want to make a walk a part of your daily routine. Maybe you want to walk for a few hours, or choose an end goal to try to achieve.

Just remember. . .steps to go on a walk:

Put one foot in front of the other (preferably outside)

That's it!

6

Pick wildflowers

There are always flowers for those who want to see them.
   —*Henri Matisse*

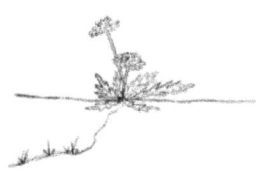

I have an old calendar page framed on my mantle with the above quote. Something that pierced my heart years ago when I didn't have the money for art, and still fills my soul with hope today.

Picking wildflowers is a two-fold experience. First there is the seeking, then there is the enjoying.

I am amazed that no matter what time of year, if I take a walk and search for blooms, I will always find them, even in the dead of winter. Finding wildflowers is a spiritual practice, a rhythm, a worship experience.

You might start out feeling despair, hopeless, even lost. But if you look you will start seeing blooms in the crack of a sidewalk, on the side of an interstate, in the bed of a rotting log. It quickly becomes a game. . .a treasure hunt that pricks at your childhood love of hide-and-seek. Searching for wildflowers is a practice in noticing, in bending down to see what is often overlooked. Wildflower walks are a great way to move your body without even knowing you're exercising.

Sometimes I just enjoy the flowers and leave them for others to notice. Other times I carefully gather a handful of what I find—delightfully mismatched and stored in old jars on my sink.

A reminder that not only will you find blooms if

you look for them, you can find that same beauty in your life; it just might be in unexpected places.

7

Play in the rain

Let the rain sing you a lullaby.

—Langston Hughes

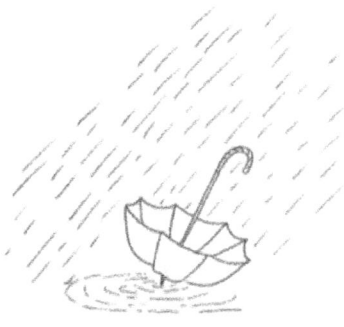

When was the last time you played in the rain? For most of us adults the answer to that question would be sometime in your childhood.

In fact, adults and their always updating weather apps are highly aware of when it's going to rain—they warn people about it, they begrudge the cancelling of outdoor activities, they over prepare.

I am not one of these people. I never know when it's going to rain and because of that, I find myself in a rain storm quite often—and with no umbrella. I always giggle because people will say something to me as I walk by them soaking wet and smiling. I just reply, "Oh! I actually have waterproof skin!" This reply always makes people stop and ponder this little fact of life.

I love the way rain feels on my skin, the way I lose my breath when it's really pouring down. I love to splash in puddles and look up into the sky and let it rinse me clean.

Next time it rains, try stepping out in it. See what happens. See if you can go long without smiling or even bursting into laughter.

There's a reason cheesy country songs have a lot of *dancing in the rain* lyrics-because it is a SENSUAL experience, an experience that fills your senses and thus your soul.

PLAY IN THE RAIN

Remember, you have water proof skin too.

8

Create without an end goal

To live a creative life, we must lose our fear of being wrong.
—*Joseph Chilton Pearce*

"I wish I was creative."

I cannot tell you how many people tell me this when I tell them I am a photographer and an author.

While I understand what they mean by this phrase, I will always adamantly disagree.

Every human is a creative being. Some people might create by decorating their home, arranging their food beautifully, making playlists for every mood, baking, or even dancing while cooking dinner.

CREATE WITHOUT AN END GOAL

Creativity does not refer to the sellability or likability of the result. Creativity is about the *process*.

I learned years ago that the key to enjoying creativity is letting go of any type of end goal. Lucky for me I am not a perfectionist. It's honestly my superpower I think. I don't mind a pile of discarded projects. I don't mind throwing out 80% of what I write. I start things without much overthinking and never look at projects as failures.

I am a terrible painter, my drawings are embarrassing, and yet I consider myself an artist. Sometimes I choose to use my well-honed skill of the camera to create photos that end up in galleries and sometimes I paint simple lines and get lost as I watch the colors blend together.

I figured out years ago that blending lines of watercolors deeply satisfied that creativity itch and kept me in a state of flow. Contrary to my work, the end result isn't astounding or memorable. Sometimes I keep these little paintings and write over the top of them with a quote or a letter to a friend. Sometimes I recycle or burn them. It does not even matter. It matters that I get pleasure from simply making them.

Lately I've really gotten into collaging; tearing out images or words from magazines that strike me and modge-podging them together to make something new—even if the new thing never sees the light of day. Even better, my little community has started hosting community collages where people can create alongside each other.

Creating is for every human. So set aside your fear of failing and break out that old sketchbook, paint some beautiful lines, or create that Spotify playlist you've been wanting to have for your morning cup. There is no wrong way to create when you show up.

CREATE WITHOUT AN END GOAL

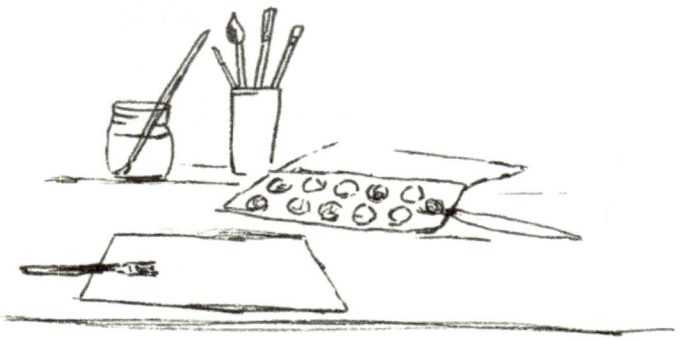

9

Watch the sun set

May every sunrise hold more promise and every sunset hold more peace.
—*Umair Siddiqui*

There are many nights I feel a pulling to my bed. A place to put my head under the covers and shut out the world. So many times I wanted to just numb out, turn on the TV and sink into my couch, but the sunset called to me. Sometimes it feels like stepping through molasses to get there but every. single. time I chose a sunset, I felt peace. Once in a while all I could do was step out of my door and crane my neck to the west, just glimpsing the edges of it all, searching for pinks and oranges.

The fact that the sun sets every single day can

make us lose track of the miracle of it. The promise that it will always come again can make us push it to the side for "another day".

Maybe you want to watch the sun set in the reflection of your kitchen window while you finish up the dishes. Maybe you want to hike to the top of a mountain and let the colors bathe you while you sip something hot or toast something bubbly. Maybe you want to have your toes in the ocean as you watch the sun dip into its endless horizon.

Don't wait for tomorrow, stay out for the sunset today.

10

Look at weird art

You can understand nothing about art, particularly modern art, if you do not understand that imagination is a value in itself.
—*Milan Kundera*

One of my favorite pleasures in visiting a new city is going to the local modern art museum. Don't get me wrong, I love a beautifully painted classic. I love the movement of Degas, the beautiful lighting of Renoir, the colors of Monet. . .but there is something about weird modern art that I absolutely delight in. I love how it makes me think, how I get to peek inside the minds of humans and their bizarre thoughts—a deep dive into the human psyche.

It's a break from things not being so damn serious. And also not so damn pretty all of the time.

When I was visiting New York City after a particularly hard season of life, I found myself in the MOMA watching a stop motion video of hot dogs dancing and racing around on a sleeping man. People were rolling their eyes walking by but I sat there laughing so hard. How brilliant that someone thought, "I would love to create something where hot dogs dance on me" Maybe it was from a dream, maybe it came from entertaining a bored toddler, but here I was being temporarily relieved from the weightiness of life and giggling on a Saturday afternoon.

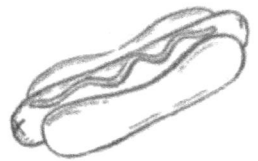

I love the unexpected. It expands my brain and makes me feel human. I love seeing a new way of looking at something.

Go to a modern art museum and find something that brings you joy. It doesn't have to make sense, be serious, or even have a point. Go with a friend and see what speaks to you and what speaks to them. Let your imagination run wild.

11

Plant something

The soil is the great connector of our lives, the source and destination of all.
　—*Wendell Berry*

I do not have a green thumb. I grew up with a mother who could grow anything and grow it well. She was always getting clippings of plants from places we visited and a year later, that plant would be growing at our home. I do not have the patience or attention to detail that it takes to be a successful gardener. Even though I know I'm not good at it, I still love getting my hands in the earth. The act of planting is the act of hoping. And the benefits are undeniable mentally and physically.

Notice this chapter does not say "plant a garden" because that would be really stressful to a good chunk of folks who read this (me included). But you don't have to plant a whole garden to experience the beauty of having your hands in the dirt.

Get your hands in the earth.

Plant some seeds or bulbs

Scatter wildflowers.

Plant a fern from the grocery story in a window box

Pull weeds from your front yard

Join a community garden

Help a neighbor spread mulch or pick up branches

Look into chaos gardening
Replant something you find on walk

This act is one of hope, not of harvest. And I believe there to be true gifts in just that.

12

Lean into the seasons

If we had not winter, the spring would not be so pleasant; if we did not sometimes taste of adversity, prosperity would not be so welcome.
—Anne Bradstreet

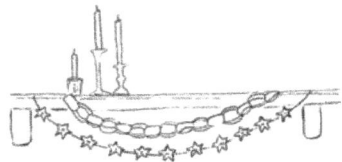

I think humans are doing a pendulum swing right now, coming back to the earth and the rhythms that unfold every year after trying to live for so many decades like seasons don't exist. Humanity has been long disconnected from this. It's evident as everyone pushes to become their best self for the new year, in the dead of winter. When you observe nature, no animals or plants or even the trees are doing anything but resting in January.

Seasonal depression is a real thing. A lot of folks struggle in the winter feeling lethargic and blue. I think that living out of harmony with nature can cause a lot of this. Of course you're going to feel blue if you're trying to get a lot done when you have the least amount of light and the least amount of energy. I used to hate winter but when I started slowing down and enjoying the rest instead of trying to "be my best self", I came to love it.

WAYS TO LEAN into the seasons:

Get outside
    Eat what is growing
    Celebrate everything
    Notice what the plants and animals are up to

. . .

LIVING in awareness of the gifts that each season brings leads to feeling connected and rooted in your life. Fall into the rhythm that comes from the earth and all the ways she changes. It will also remind us, after a long hard season, that there is an end and a new one will always begin.

13

Welcome Spring

It is spring again. The earth is like a child that knows poems by heart.
—*Rainer Maria Rilke*

Thanks to winter there is not a soul on earth who doesn't squeal when they see the first sunshine yellow daffodil popping through the earth. Spring is a miracle that I will never get over. New life is the name of the game and I always feel like I am also coming to life. With the new life I feel a shedding of the old. I want to clean my home, donate things I don't use, and throw open the doors to let in the breeze.

Unlike this capitalist society's push for new years resolutions, THIS is the time to make goals.

Spring activities to lean into:
    Clean your house

    Collect wildflowers and bring them inside—

    Make some goals

    Start new habits

    Run barefoot in the grass

    Have a picnic

    Paint outside

    Give things away that you don't need

    CREATE

14

Welcome Summer

Live in the sunshine. Swim in the sea. Drink in the wild air.
　—*Ralph Waldo Emerson*

Summer is a container for memories. The long days give so much opportunity for adventure and fellowship. Nature is teeming with so much going on that we tend to spend our time outside: swimming, hiking, playing freeze tag, surrounded by fireflies at dusk.

I, personally, struggle with how my body feels in summer with the heat, but I've learned that standing in a river several times a week allows me to manage just fine. I love summer because there are more opportunities to be with people. Vacations and lack of school give so much more space to connect. . .and sometimes over really yummy food.

Summer activities to lean into:
Get in water
Be with people
Have a picnic
Stay outside after dark (because fireflies are basically fairies)
Sleep in
Take every opportunity for an adventure
Be in nature
Eat all the yummy foods that summer brings

15

Welcome Fall

I'm so glad I live in a world where there are Octobers.
—*L. M. Montgomery*

I relish the fall. The colors of the changing leaves, the crisp air that beckons some of my favorite memories, and the start of a cozy season. I swear, some of the magic of fall goes back to the new start of school as a child and the joy of getting a Lisa Frank notebook or a new dress. Fall is a time to embrace change—a time to welcome the break from the long, busy, hot days of summer.

Take note from the trees and let go of what doesn't serve you, so that you will have a season of new growth.

Autumn activities to lean into:

Enjoy warm things like soup and cider

Slow down

Gather fall leaves and press them between wax paper with an iron (and then tape it to your windows)

Eat root veggies

Build bonfires on the short evenings

Embrace change

Get cozy

Let go of what no longer serves you

16

Welcome Winter

Winter is a lingering season, it is a time to gather golden moments, embark upon a sentimental journey, and enjoy every idle hour.
—*John Boswell*

I used to hate winter. In fact, I think most people think they hate winter. Seasonal depression disorder skyrockets in those short, harsh months. There's lots of things to hate about it if you're trying to live the way that you live in the summer.

Winter is a gift. Winter is a gift of pause, rest, and reflection. When I started learning about the cultures that live in the harshest of winters, I learned I was doing winter wrong. I was trying to be productive. New Years resolutions of a new me when my body was saying "NOPE. I want to sleep more and move less" were making it worse.

Now, winter is about bringing light into the darkness, resting deeply without guilt, crafting-reading-writing, reflecting on the past year WITHOUT goals. It's beautiful.

Winter is now my favorite.

WINTER ACTIVITIES TO LEAN INTO:
Rest
Light candles
Journal and reflect
Go to bed early
Pick up a hobby to occupy your hands
Walk outside even if it's cold
Rest in who you are, you only have to *be*

17

Take a bath

There must be quite a few things that a hot bath won't cure, but I don't know many of them.
—*Sylvia Plath*

I agree with Sylvia. Hot baths are my safe place. It's where I do my thinking, or sometimes my not thinking. It's where I cry, where I let myself *feel*. Maybe it's because we are made up of over 60% water, maybe it is the fact that for 9 months we grow in water, but there is something primal and comforting about being in warm water.

In a lot of other countries there are community rituals surrounding bathing: Korean bath houses, Turkish baths, German health spas. I went to my first communal bath house in Japantown in San Francisco in my 20s and I was hooked. It was sacred and unashamed and it felt like coming home to be in that echoey chamber of women just simply taking a bath.

A lot of times baths are only shown as a luxurious splurge. Saved only for people with all the time and all the money. You probably are picturing something like this right now: a woman with a mountain of bubbles, holding a champagne, surrounded by candles everywhere, and smelling of roses.

Once in a while I will take a fancy bath with flowers and scents, but mostly I keep it simple.

Some people are disgusted with the idea of baths and to them I would say, take a shower instead. Or even take a shower and THEN take a bath. Either gives a break, a place to drown out the regular daily chatter. A chance to reset, to literally rinse the day off of you.

Taking a bath is my number one most used tool to feel better, to change my energy, or my day.

Do it how you like! Make it pretty, make it smell good, save a special drink for it. Or be like me and just GET IN and let everything melt away.

TAKE A BATH

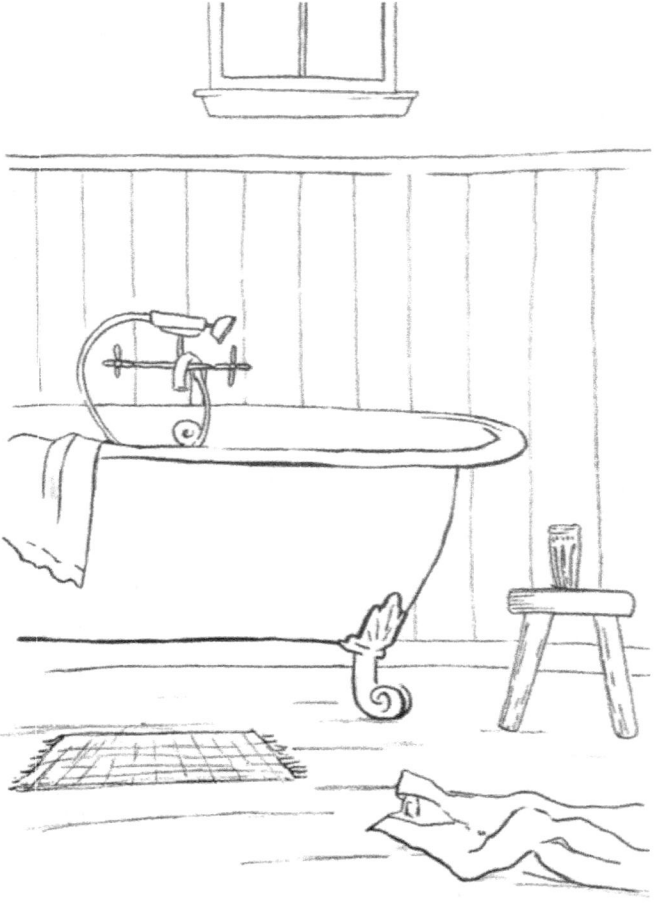

18

Go to the theatre

I regard the theatre as the greatest of all art forms, the most immediate way in which a human being can share with another the sense of what it is to be a human being.
—*Oscar Wilde*

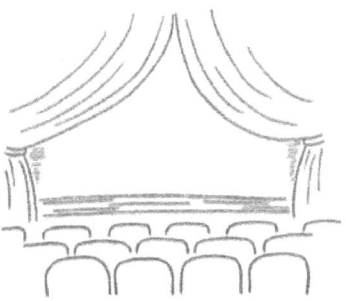

GO TO THE THEATRE

With streaming services delivering thousands of entertaining movies and shows to your couch at the press of a button, we are entirely drowning in options to enthrall our minds. And yet the dwindling option of watching live theatre is still there, offering you a collective and deeply human experience that will satisfy something deep in your soul.

Most people forget what a thrill it is to watch something unfold on a stage and experience it with other people. The nuanced energy brought on by certain actors, even the small mistakes make for a very delightful experience.

Maybe you want to save and splurge on a musical on Broadway with a live orchestra and fantastical costumes. Maybe you want to see the local theatre put on something thought provoking and new. Maybe you want to go to the local High School's production of Annie just to dip your toes in the pond of trying something new. Maybe you want to see the Nutcracker ballet at Christmas like you did when you were a child.

Get dressed up, get excited, file into the theatre seats, put your phone on airplane mode, and feel the energy that is building in anticipation of the show. Enjoy an experience that will wake up your senses and remind you of the special privilege of being alive.

19

Slow down

If a man does not keep pace with his companions, perhaps it is because he hears a different drummer. Let him step to the music which he hears, however measured or far away.
—*Thoreau*

Have you ever said to yourself, "I just want to move to a little cabin in the woods."? Or is that just me?

Our culture is one of fast paced work, ultra productive driven days, traffic, social media advertising, and a general sense of *we aren't doing enough* even though we are doing more than ever.

Most of us will not go all Henry David Thoreau and actually move to a cabin in the woods, but there absolutely are benefits to slowing down your pace of life. We can visit that *cabin* even just for a few moments whenever we want.

You might immediately think of STOPPING, like sitting on the porch or meditating. But slowing down is not that.

It's finding tenderness in the space, a rhythmic hum that can move you into a lovely trance.

Sometimes I do this by doing "farm chores" like I would if I didn't live in the age of shiny appliances. Washing dishes by hand is actually very soothing to me. The sound of the water and the warmth of having my hands in it lull me into a place of meditation. Even though I have a perfectly working dishwasher to my left, I still like to meditate at the sink. Building a fire, stitching a button back on, or rolling bees wax candles can all be tools to bring us to a space that we just don't enter in often. That rhythmic state of doing, just slower.

Sometimes I slow down by shutting off my phone and putting a record on. Simply the act of choosing one from my collection, letting it slip out of its sleeve, and listening to the entire thing feels good. It makes life seem temporarily manageable. Of course I have a smart phone that I can tell to play any song in the world from across the room, and that is 95% of how I listen to music, but playing a record every once in a while is a treat and a reminder.

Maybe you dip your toes into slower living one choice at a time—sprinkled here and there, maybe you find that in those moments your body sighs "YES! This is what we need" and you make drastic changes in order to live more intentionally and slowly.

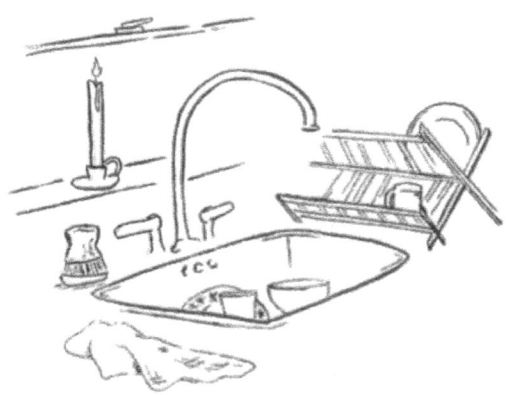

20

Say nice things to yourself

Talk to yourself like you would to someone you love.
—Brené Brown

Having a daughter changed me. It's the strangest experience to have an outside look into the journey of growing up, to hear feelings I had as a child come out of her lips. Words like "I'm so ugly," or "I'm so stupid." Remembering how I felt those same things and how fresh they were, mixed with how much I loved this child, how beautiful and smart and special she was, I started talking to myself the way I talk to my daughter or to a friend.

Sometimes I think of the words, sometimes I say them out loud when I'm looking in the mirror, and sometimes I write them out and put them somewhere obvious.

I am a beautiful creation
Your body is strong and perfect
I love the way that you always find hope.

Being a demanding bully to ourselves might feel like the normal thing to do in this day and age, but we can change this. We can say nice things to ourselves even if it feels cringy and odd. It is not self-centered or self- indulgent to take notice of the good things that make us who we are . Bonus points, our children and neighbors and friends and even our parents might pick up on it.

4 years after starting to talk to myself kindly, I walked into my preteen daughter's bathroom and saw a little sign she painted that said "I like myself." May we all come to like ourselves.

Talk to yourself like you would someone you love and watch it change everything.

21

Sit by a tree

All our wisdom is stored in the trees.
—*Santosh Kalwar*

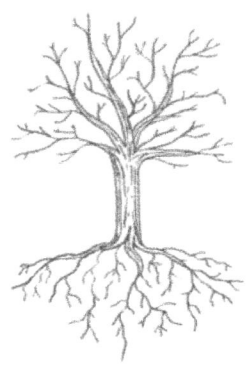

SIT BY A TREE

I've been drawn to trees ever since I can remember. At the age of four I would find myself at the bottom of the tall ones with my chin pressed against the rough bark, looking up till I got dizzy. In my childhood in the southeast, I would run and climb the thick ancient oak trees when I felt misunderstood and rest in the crooks of branches. As a teenager I walked barefoot in the fields, admiring the buds of baby leaves about to sprout; as a young mother I clung to the exposed roots next to the river and sighed with relief as my fingers sank into the soil.

Trees are living breathing souls. I can't tell you how often I sit at the base of them and feel the strength of their roots under me as well as their hope stretching to the heavens above me.

There is undeniable power there and simply by sitting near them, I feel renewed.

Maybe you live near forests that are rich with beckoning adventures and trees of every size. Maybe you have a sapling at the corner of your lot and it's all you can do to muster the energy to sit next to it.

Look up and feel small, feel the roots that you can't see that keep this tree from topping over in a storm, and imagine yourself with roots to ground you and leaves to stretch and grow.

22

Work outdoors

Chop your own wood and it will warm you twice.
　—*Henry Ford*

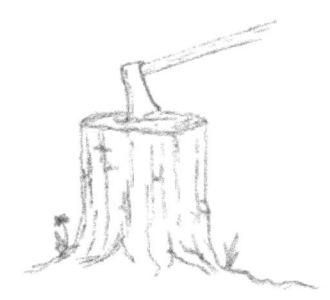

When 2020 came and the world shut down, my quarantine activity of choice was chopping wood. It became a ritual and soon became a lifeline. I would go onto my land and gather downed branches. I would drag big ones and gather arms full of smaller ones and take them to the chopping block. I would then spend an hour chopping them into the perfect size to make a fire and then would enjoy stacking them.

Being outside, doing something physically challenging and accomplishing it was the perfect combination to pull me outside of myself and the doomsday feeling that life presented at that time.

We do not get enough outside work time. We simply do not. And I think that has a lot to do with our rising depression, our inability to go to sleep, and our restlessness. But we can't all be farmers.

So play around with outdoor work. Pick a project, plant something, clear your garden bed, even try chopping wood if you're like me.

Just because we don't have to do it anymore doesn't mean that it isn't good for us. Accomplishing something outside and going to sleep that night feeling proud of yourself will change how you feel. And if you keep it up, it will change your life.

23

Wear something that makes you smile

Life is too short to wear boring clothes.
—*Carly Cushnie*

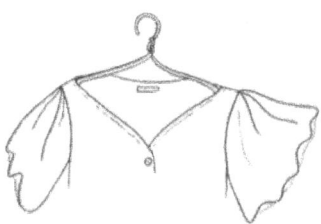

A lot of our days are spent pleasing people, even from deciding what to wear first thing in the morning.

We wear things that make us look the thinnest and show off our best features. Or only wearing something in eternal autumn or whatever color wheel someone locked you in at a mall somewhere last year. If we aren't trying to please people, we are often just dressing in what's comfortable, especially in seasons of depression. Sweats and comfy t-shirts become a literal uniform sometimes. Or sometimes it is literally armor.

I remember one day deciding I was going to wear a dress I know didn't flatter me. It hung wrong and wasn't trending, but oh my goodness did it make me happy. The swish of the material around my legs, the colors that felt like they were awake and joyful. Wearing that dress brought confidence to me, and a genuine joy that made people notice me that day. The ripple effect of choosing to wear something that brought me joy was much bigger than I would have thought. By the end of the day I had talked to so many people, smiled so much, and felt beautiful all day long.

A dear friend, Andrea, who was struggling with depression decided to wear something that made her happy every single day and document it on Tik-Tok.

Months later, not only was she looking beautiful and vibrant, she was falling in love with her future husband, adopting a dog, and finding a reason to smile every day.

Clothes are powerful, transformational tools that we have access to every day.

Put on that skirt that makes you smile, even if it doesn't match anything. Wear those shoes, slip on the shirt that brings you joy, dress up even though no one else is.

24

Take yourself on a date

You're always with yourself, so you might as well enjoy the company.
—Diane von Furstenberg

One cold December day, I found myself alone near Christmas. My 17 year marriage had ended and my children were with their dad that evening. The busyness of the holiday season felt like it was worlds away from me. I found myself standing downtown watching happy families laugh as they shopped and I glanced through the restaurant windows at cozy couples gazing at each other over cocktails. This feeling I was observing, one of coziness and warmth felt like it was so far out of reach. I mentally ran through a list of my friends I could invite to dinner but I knew all of them were with their children doing something festive. All of a sudden I was struck with a wild idea and I decided to take myself on a date then and there. I wasn't dressed for it, but I found myself at the bar at the fanciest restaurant in town. I ordered a holiday cocktail and a side of broccoli. I sat up straight and let the hum of the place surround me with warmth. I chatted with the couple next to me, I made friends with the waitress, and I smiled for two hours straight.

That night was powerful for me. It taught me that I don't have to wait for connection and coziness. That I can step into it any time I please.

Take yourself on a date, try the dessert, smile at everyone around you. This is a privilege not a pity party. You don't have to wait for anyone.

TAKE YOURSELF ON A DATE

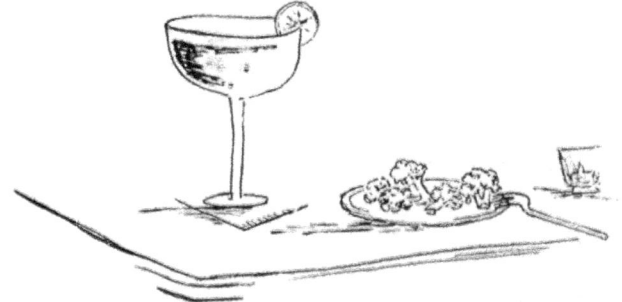

25

Help someone

There is no exercise better for the heart than reaching down and lifting people up.
—*John Holmes*

There is something transformational about helping someone. Even if I'm in a hard season myself, taking a moment to get outside of my reality to lift someone up can majorly shift how things feel. It can be small, like tipping a tired barista extra or large, like showing up to someone's house to help with cleaning after they have a baby. It's not about the action as much as it is about taking a break from centering your world around yourself and putting your energy outwards.

If you've dealt with times of depression, like me, you are probably actually an expert on ways you can lift someone else up. You know how the smallest gesture can make you feel seen and important. How just a little action can change around your week.

Ideas to get you started:
-Give someone a genuine compliment
-Pay for someone's lunch
-Pick flowers for your mom
-Bring in your neighbor's trash can
-Take your niece to ice cream
-Go watch a movie with someone who is lonely
-Wash dishes
-Listen to a friend
-Buy a co-worker their favorite snack
-Adopt a child at Christmas

100 drops of water

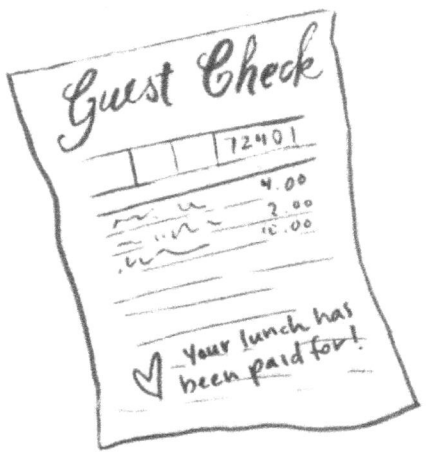

26

Light a candle

Learn to light a candle in the darkest moments of someone's life.
—Roy T. Bennett

For the longest time I had candles sitting around my home gathering dust. I got them for my wedding and they sat on my mantle for years—through multiple moves, yet never being lit. Candles are oftentimes saved for "something special" and thus, rarely or never used. We save them for "one day," but that day never comes.

A few years into motherhood when the days were endlessly long, I started using candles for every day dinners. I'd light them over styrofoam takeout containers or simple hot dogs. I would sometimes light them in my room for a few minutes when I was feeling bleak. In an instant, everything is a little more elevated, a little more magical. I learned to embrace the wax on the table as a sign that our life was romantic because we CHOSE for it to be romantic.

Candles bring light into shadows and dance around like darkness is nothing. They bathe everyone in what feels like moonlight.

I prefer non-scented tapered candles which I switch out from thrifted candle stick holders. I love the way they daintily flicker and slowly drip down the sides.

What I really love is marking the ordinary as special with this simple little ritual. Make your day romantic and light a candle!

LIGHT A CANDLE

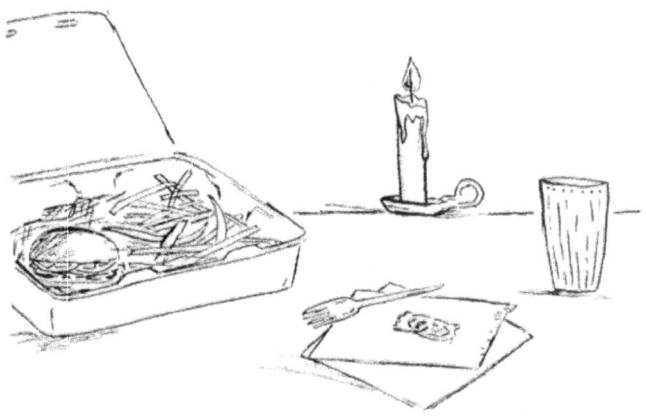

27

Pick up treasures

It is perhaps a more fortunate destiny to have a taste for collecting shells than to be born a millionaire.
   —*Robert Louis Stevenson*

PICK UP TREASURES

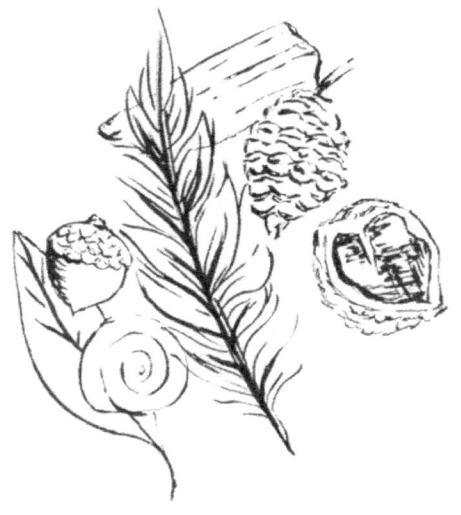

Do you remember what it felt like to be a child and to find treasures outside? Maybe a rock that looked like it might be gold, a feather you found in a bush, a piece of wood shaped like a heart? Why did we ever stop searching for treasures in our daily lives?

I think many adults are jolted back into the wonder of looking for treasures when they go on vacation at the beach and find themselves with nothing but time to comb the edge of the water for shells that catch their eye. I love sitting on the beach and watching adults engrossed in the hunt.

I say looking for treasures every day should be the antidote to the harshness of adulting. A gift we give ourselves every single day.

Pick up the stones, the lucky pennies, the fallen bird's nest, the leaf that looks like it was painted (even if you know that it will wither by the next day). Make piles above your sink, fill jars and empty them after a year.

My home is layered with art, family heirlooms, and treasures. I have a piece of driftwood from my favorite day at the beach with my children, smooth glass I found at the river, feathers I collected on walks. I love them because they remind me that there is beauty everywhere. And that all we need to do is look.

28

Skinny dip

And a softness came from the starlight and filled me to the bone.
—*W.B. Yeats*

There is something holy about slipping into water with nothing separating you from it. All of a sudden you are suspended—a returning to the first feelings of being held in a womb. I remember the summer I convinced my Great Aunt Lucy to let me go into the ocean after dark, naked as the day I was born. I had read about skinny dipping in a book and was delighted with the thought of being free. The feeling I felt slipping into the warm, salty water under a brilliant starry sky felt like home. The way the water enveloped me satiated a soul hunger I had felt since I had consciousness.

Ever since that night, floating on my back sandwiched by the sky and the water always brings me back.

If the thought of public nudity absolutely terrifies you, I have found sensory deprivation tanks or float tanks to be a very close relative to skinny dipping as you float on salt water away from onlookers.

Maybe you will run into an icy mountain stream and return pink cheeked and giggling–life force pumping through your veins like never before. Maybe you'll slip into a pool in the wee morning hours and float until you feel lulled into rest. Maybe you will slip your bathing suit off under the waves of the ocean and smile as your body melts into the water that connects us all. Just your little secret.

SKINNY DIP

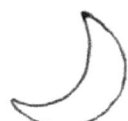

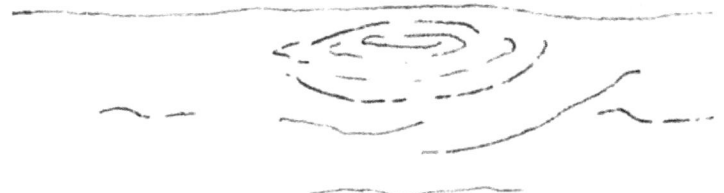

29

Join a group

We all want to feel a sense of belonging. This isn't a character flaw. It's fundamental to the human experience. Our finest achievements are possible when people come together to work for a common cause. School spirit, the rightful pride we feel in our community, our heritage, our religion, and our families, all come from the value we place on belonging to a group.
—Rosalind Wiseman

I saw a documentary recently that really inspired me called *Join or Die*. In it they went over the very interesting history of people joining groups and how that trend is falling more and more every day.

Some of the perks of joining a club are of course to not feel alone, and also surprisingly it's being with folks different than you. We have gotten used to hanging with people just like us and because of that we are missing out on a huge flavor of life and a huge skill of having our world expanded with different people from different walks of life.

I've been in some clubs in my lifetime and I can look back and feel such happiness about those times in my life. Showing up with other people to connect over something is powerful. I've been in mom groups, book clubs, dance classes, grief circles, and co-working spaces to name a few.

Take a look around your community and see if there's anything that sparks your interest. I'm sure they would love you to show up and bring your own personal magic to the table. Book clubs are easy to join and give you a great excuse to read (which is a wonderful grounding skill).

I think the key to the whole thing being successful is:

- Show up (don't let yourself make excuses)
- Be open and be yourself
- Allow others to do the same

30

Pour a cup of tea

There is no trouble so great or grave that cannot be diminished by a nice cup of tea.
—*Bernard Paul Heroux*

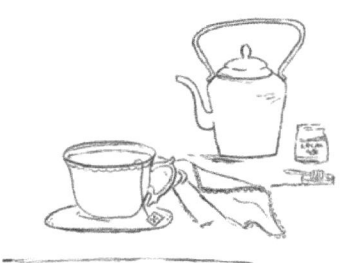

POUR A CUP OF TEA

Something I wish we Americans had kept from our English heritage is the ritual of tea. I grew up with a grandmother who always paused for tea. Sometimes we donned big sun hats and feasted on a dozen little delicacies, sometimes it was just a warm cup on an afternoon that needed a little magic in it. I remember a normal Thursday being brought to life with the toasting of some bread, some butter, and honey. The ordinary became extraordinary in the name of tea. The beauty of tea is in the rest, not in the details.

Cultures that give space for a tea ritual are onto something. My US culture's ritual is a hurried cup of overpriced coffee in a Starbucks drive through in the afternoon slump and we are missing out.

Maybe tea sounds like a watered down and out of date beverage, but upon just the tiniest bit of stepping into it—you will find that the slowing down, even just to boil the water, is a gift. Invite a friend over for a cup, experiment on trying different kinds in that witching hour of work in which times seems to slow down to a painful pace. Plan an event for friends and go all out.

Tea gives space for connection with others, with rest, with every day magic that we so need to infuse our lives with.

31

Sifting

Tidying is the act of confronting yourself.
　—*Marie Kondō*

There is a mood I get in sometimes... antsy would probably be the closest word that matches what that energy feels like. It's a feeling that wants to move but maybe is ping-ponging all over the place. What I found helps reinstate me to homeostasis is any kind of sifting. Going through an old drawer and putting things where they belong, walking the aisles of an antique store and finding something you like, purging old greeting cards, going through your toppling side table book stack. Sifting is mediation.

One time my life was literally falling apart. I was

getting divorced, a large hole under the sink of my rental house had let in an entire village of woodland rats, and I had 12 dollars to my name. It felt pretty bad, pretty lay down on the ground and give up sort of bad. And yet, I found my way to a drawer in the yellow dresser I had salvaged and painted that Summer. It was so full of junk and mismatched cards that you couldn't even open it. That drawer represented my life; chaos, broken, unfixable.

Piece by piece I laid out each thing on my floor. I sifted everything slowly. Keep, recycle, donate, trash. I married cards with envelopes and started making beauty out of the mess. When I was done, my house still needed defending from the rats, I was still getting divorced, but somehow it didn't feel as daunting.

Thrifting is my favorite way to sift. I will slip into a thrift store before school pickup and spend 10 minutes combing the sweaters for the perfect non-itchy wool one in just the color I like. I will scour the shelves of nicknacks to find a tiny bowl with a bird on it to put my earrings in. Very often I do not even buy anything and emerge just feeling calmer. Thrifting without high pressure to find something is a little treat to your nervous system.

. . .

FIND something that feels like too much and make sense of it. Maybe this is by tracing the edges of the dresses at the local thrift store or righting your junk drawer. Take your time, get into a zone, enjoy.

32

Write a letter by hand

Letter writing is the only device combining solitude with good company.
—Lord Byron

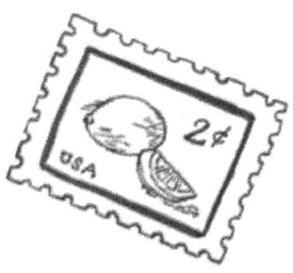

In my line of work, I have found myself many times helping people sort through their memorabilia: old photos all curled at the edges, sea glass from their honeymoon, movie ticket stubs, and lots and lots of letters. I've noticed the younger my clients are the less they have any letters to save and treasure. Sadly, the coming generations will not have many letters to keep even though they are almost constantly in communication on their phones.

Handwritten letters are a lost art. While writing letters for everything isn't practical, I don't feel like it needs to become a lost art. We can still take opportunities to indulge in this meditative practice. Letter writing is a creative process with no right or wrong way. The act of taking the time to arrange your words in a slow, intentional way will absolutely shift things for you. Maybe your heart rate will lower, you might feel more embodied or present. Your mind might feel gratitude for the gift of letting yourself focus for a while on something that isn't flashing or advertising to you. Something that will make you feel good but will also make someone else feel thought of and seen.

Maybe you want to go Jo March on your letter: a quill pen, a lit candle, and romantic music swelling in the background. Maybe you collect little cards that get you started with being perfectly designed for a particular friend.

You can write a letter to:

Your mom

Your postman

Your neighbor, best friend, lover, child, or barista

You can write to people you've lost contact with (like your 5th grade teacher or your childhood best friend)

You can write to people you talk to every day

Letters are special in that they will give you joy twice. Once when you write it and another time when the recipient receives it.

33

Make your bed

The secret to getting ahead is getting started.
—*Mark Twain*

Making my bed has never been a habit that has stuck with me. Something about knowing I will undo it in half a day's time makes me feel like I am saving precious minutes by leaving the blanket and sheets in disarray.

If you're into the self-help world, making your bed is often talked about. These guru books taunt me with the fact that this one task will automatically propel me into the life of my dreams and yet I still don't do it every day.

Despite my rejection of this tip for success, on mornings when I wake up and stare at the day ahead and it feels really, really hard…maybe even impossible, I make my bed. Something about making order out of chaos right there at the start gives me the tiniest boost to get out of my bed and keep going. As the day progresses I'm less tempted to fall back into the comfort of my covers.

It's simple but it's infinitely powerful. I tend to sabotage myself here because it's too simple. I will start thinking that I can make my bed **AFTER** I purchase all organic cotton sheets and a comforter that costs more than a car payment-that to make a bed it needs to be pretty.

Repeat after me…"I don't need anything to make my bed. I just need to mark that the day has started by doing something different."

Regardless if you become a bed maker or not, indulge in being the kind of person who makes their bed, because **YOU ARE!**

100 drops of water

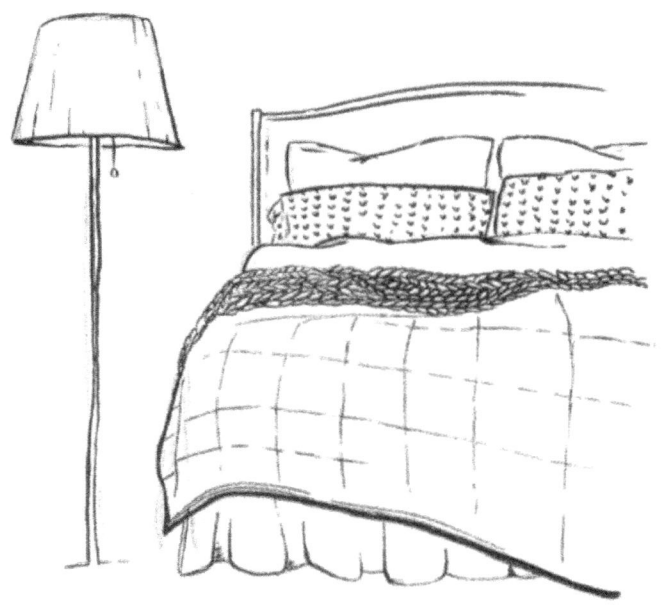

34

Watch the sun rise

Even the darkest night will end and the sun will rise.
—Hugo

I have two friends who are sunrise people. When I'm on a trip or vacation with them, no matter what happened the night before, you will find them facing east come sunrise. If you were to type sunrise into the search bar on their phone, hundreds of images would pop up, showing their delight in this daily event.

I've always deeply felt that I am not *a sunrise kind of a person*. I love to sleep too much. I am frequently depressed and reluctant to wake up from a state in which life doesn't seem so heavy. Sunrises were not for me.

For years I observed these friends coming back

from their sunrise viewings. It felt like upon their return, they would be glowing like they had just seen something holy. And they had…the birth of a day. It took me leaving a marriage that was draining every ounce of life energy from me to get me to a place where I wanted what they were experiencing on those early mornings.

I have now been to many a sunrise, and have found myself in awe—transformed by the experience. I thought that the point of watching the sun rise was simply to appreciate the beauty of the colors that unfold. I found instead that I was drawn to the darkness before it, the holding of my breath till I saw that first golden edge starting to warm the world. I found incredible comfort in the fact that no matter what–the sun will rise; no matter who is elected into office, if I have a job, if I take a day off from the grind of daily life, the sun is there, ushering in a new day.

Maybe you want to gather a thermos of something delicious and hot and drive in the wee morning hours to a place with vast views.

Maybe you stand with your nose pressed against the cold glass of your window, straining to see the first hints of a new day.

Maybe you wake up early and it's so cloudy you

don't see much and yet the magic, the stillness of a new morning ignites you.

Maybe you decide you want to greet the sun every single day as a ritual that connects you to the order of the universe.

Whether you watch the sun rise once or a hundred times, it will never leave you the same.

35

Learn something new

Live as if you were to die tomorrow. Learn as if you were to live forever.
—*Mahatma Gandhi*

I know I might be in the minority here, but I miss school. There is nothing like the feeling of sitting in class with a blank notebook and a pen perched on the surface ready to take notes about something I didn't know about. When I was 13, I figured out I could research on the internet and would spend hours blissfully diving into any subject I wanted to know more about. Not because it was assigned, but because I was hungry to know more.

In our society learning is so often a burden and it stops when you finally achieve the level of education you're after. But we were created to continue learning and growing.

It is such a gift to myself to sit down and watch a documentary about something I'm curious about, to take my grown self to a museum, to read a biography about someone I want to know more about. The gift is in two parts.

Not only does it feel good to take a break from the grind or the scroll and do something new, it helps me to step back and see a bigger picture of the world and where I fit in. Learning always inspires me.

Maybe you treat yourself to a documentary in place of your usual tv show. Maybe you take a trip to immerse yourself into the museums around your small town. Maybe you decide to take up a new hobby that you can fit in after the kids are in bed—one in which you will find inspiring podcasts or articles on to keep on learning.

Learning is a gift, not a chore, and rearranging that in your brain can provide a lifetime of fulfillment and growth.

100 drops of water

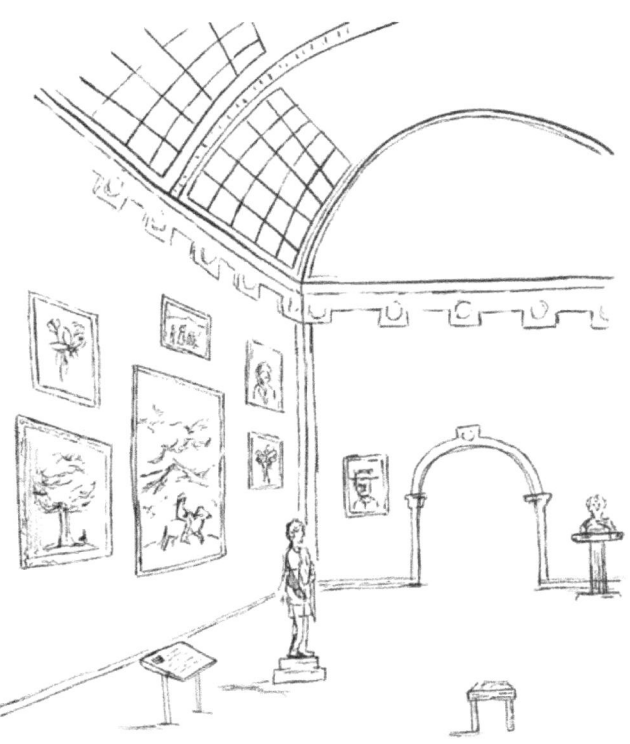

36

Check something off

Everything is hard before it is easy.
—*Goethe*

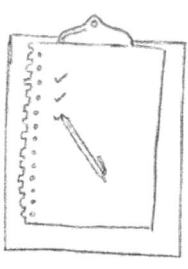

The random tasks we carry around in our subconscious can feel like way too much to hold. Mental load is a thing. For me it's mailing things, calling customer service, taxes, and insurance. For several of my best friends it is things like hanging photos on the wall, making an album, or planning a birthday party. Regardless of what feels hard to you, taking the time to do what you've been putting off, can drastically lighten how you feel.

In those times when we aren't so well, it is easy for little things to pile up and get pushed to the side. But not doing them doesn't mean they aren't still there in the corners of our mind, reminding us that we are failing.

Since Covid, our culture has leaned heavily into the self-care/mental health day. What used to be something that was unheard of is now part of regular life. I'm not saying that's a bad thing. Of course rest and reset are important, but we cannot take mental health days all the time without suffering in the long term. We also have to do boring, hard, cumbersome tasks in order to keep enjoying life.

Doing something that has been nagging at you for however long, will absolutely make you feel better. Not only will you feel better, you might recognize how much easier it was than what you had built up in your head. You might even wonder why in the world you hadn't just done it before so you could have your brain corners back.

Doing that task (you probably already know what it is) and completing it will also
1. Put you in the category of "People who get shit done"
2. Snowball into more productivity so that you can get back to enjoying life instead of hiding from your to-do list.

Pick one small thing you've been dreading and do it.

- Set a timer for 10 minutes—you can do anything for 10 minutes. And sometimes it doesn't even take 10 minutes to do the thing you've been dreading.
- Check in with how you feel when you complete something. Remember this feeling of accomplishment and how long it took to feel it.

37

Dance

We should consider every day lost in which we have not danced at least once.
—*Friedrich Wilhelm Nietzsche*

Bodies are incredible self-healing vessels.

At 36 I found myself separated from my husband of 17 years and starting over. My body had shut down for so long that even walking a few hundred feet exhausted me. I felt like my life was over. No amount of therapy, positive meditation, or journaling would fix what felt permanently broken.

In a way, my body had protected me for years by staying in fight, flight, or freeze mode. I was in a dissociated state for my entire life because of things I couldn't control. Not being in my body allowed me to stay in places that harmed me. What I didn't know was that my body could heal itself and it could heal quickly. All I had to do was dance.

I showed up to my first dance class stiff, awkward, and definitely wearing the wrong outfit. I had gained so much weight and seeing myself in the mirror felt like…that woman wasn't me.

I didn't go to dance to get back into my body. I went because my empty rental house was too much on that Saturday morning. But what a happy accident to find myself there. Dancing that day trickled into the fastest, most glorious healing of my body and soul. I started doing it every Monday and before I knew it I was spending more and more time in my own body. I was moving through grief and not keeping it in. I was changing my inner voice to one that believed in myself. Soon I was dancing every day.

Being embodied and moving your body regularly will change your life. And the terrific thing is that anyone can do it, anywhere, for free.

This past summer I stopped going to my dance class for a few months to save money. It didn't seem like a big deal because I felt mostly healed. I plummeted into severe depression and lost hold of my embodiment so quickly. I now keep dancing in the same category that I do my medicine. Necessary.

Maybe you're haunted by that middle school dance in which you DID NOT KNOW WHAT TO DO WITH YOUR HANDS. Maybe you grew up dancing but in a way that was all about performance and perfection.

I invite you to shed what you think dance is. Turn on a song you like in the darkness of your own home and just move your body. No one will see, and if the lights are out, you will not even see. It might feel so silly you can't even finish it.

Keep going.

That's it.

Even if you hated the experience, you might notice immediate changes in your body—a warmth, a fullness. Do it again. Soon your brain will stop trying to trick you into stopping with its list of reasons you shouldn't. Dancing is a nervous system massage.

Maybe you're going to "awkward dance" with your kids, maybe you want to get into classes to learn more and have something consistent. Maybe you'll find you love dancing in a group or with a partner. Maybe you go to a free dance in the middle of the woods or maybe you want to perform burlesque one day. Maybe you'll just shake it for 5 minutes on gloomy days when you can't get out of your funk.

Don't let anyone take this free medicine from you.

38

Host a party

This is the power of gathering: it inspires us, delightfully, to be more hopeful, more joyful, more thoughtful: in a word, more alive.
—Alice Waters

100 drops of water

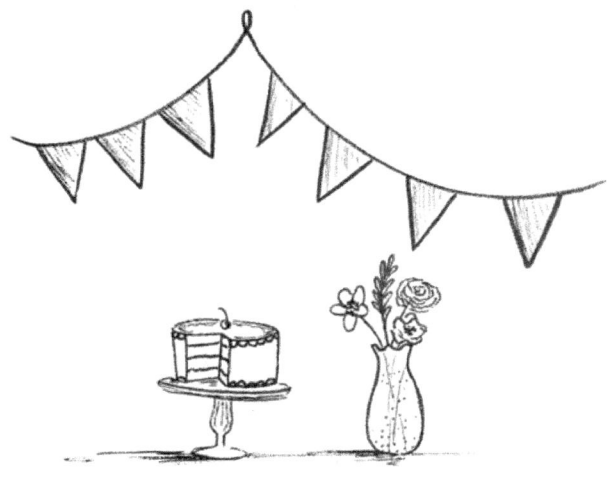

When was the last time you went to a party? I'd venture to say most adults don't go to parties regularly. I used to be so mad that movies and books from pre-1960s all contained fabulous parties, balls, and dances. The only parties I found myself at were awkward kid parties where I had to small talk with parents while gnawing on the hardest piece of pizza ever. When I turned 30 I realized that I probably was never going to be invited to a grande ball and so I decided to throw one myself. It wasn't hard. I just spoke it into being, had a fun dress made, and moved the furniture in my living room. I had friends bring a dish to share, hooked up a speaker and blasted a nice mix of Celtic fiddle tunes and early 2000's club music. The result was a night just like I had always envisioned. I got to dress up, twirl, chat in the corner with friends, and laugh until 1:00 am.

For a while there, I hosted a ball every year around the holidays. Then I moved into a cozy era and my parties were smaller and we wore pajamas.

I think sometimes we adults can feel left out, we can feel like everyone else is doing things and we aren't. But hosting a party (any kind of party you want) puts you in the driver's seat and gives you the opportunity to be the creator of whatever kind of party you desire.

Maybe you want to invite friends over to paint and drink tea. Maybe you want to throw a dance and make it fancy. Maybe you want to host a regular monthly gig with themes. You could have it catered, you could do a potluck, you could spend a week cooking if that's your thing. It doesn't have to be perfect, it doesn't even have to include a lot of guests, it doesn't even have to make sense to anyone else. This is a way to find your people, to create memories and traditions, to invite others into celebration and festivities.

The sky is the limit.

Party ideas-
    Craft/PJ party
    Full moon bonfire
    Decade cookout
    Renaissance Ball
    Garden Tea party
    90's block party
    Fancy Oscar's viewing party
    Rent a bounce house because adulting is hard —party

39

Forest bathing

Going to the woods is going home.
　—John Muir

100 drops of water

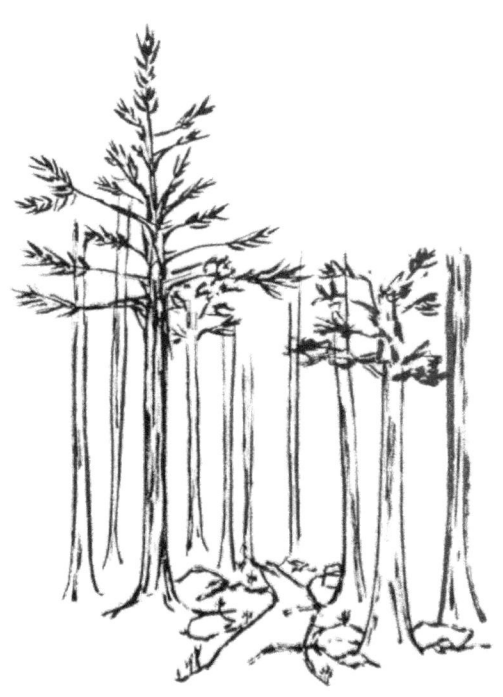

FOREST BATHING

I heard the term *forest bathing* a few years ago and LOVED it. Even though I have been forest bathing since I can remember, I never had a word for it. The feeling of newness I get after being in the woods does feel like a bath. The kind of bath that is long, warm, and maybe with a drippy candle perched on the side of the tub. The kind of bath that gives you rest in your bones.

I get the same feeling washing over me as when I walk through woods, letting the dappled sunlight through the branches lull me into a trance.

There is so much research about trees and their healing powers. Not only do they give us our oxygen, their bodies (both decaying and growing) provide incredible regenerative properties. The stillness that you feel in a grove of trees that is actually teeming with life, calms my spirit.

I frequently fantasize about living in the woods. That hasn't quite worked out for me yet, but even 20 minutes in the woods every few days keeps me sane. Sometimes I walk for miles in silence. Sometimes I make it to the edge and sit amongst the giants, enjoying the feeling of being small.

Forest bathing is simple and free. Walk into the woods—you don't have to do or be anything—let the forest bathe you in its magic.

40

Play a favorite album

Music acts like a magic key, to which the most tightly closed heart opens.
　—*Maria Augusta von Trapp*

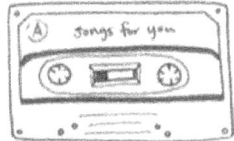

PLAY A FAVORITE ALBUM

I love streaming music. I love discovering new music, playing any song under the sun, mixing genres, or playing playlists based on my moods. But I do miss the experience of getting a new CD and listening to it all the way through. I miss the familiar feelings I would get when my mom put in our old Asleep at the Wheel cassette tape on road trips.

Sometimes it's nice to play a familiar album and let it transport you; sing every word, don't skip any songs. For me, there are a few albums from the 90s and every time I listen to them I am instantly hit with the energy of feeling young. Sometimes I listen to albums I listened to when I was sad and I am instantly reminded how far I've come. Vivaldi's four seasons reminds me of Thanksgiving growing up. James Taylor makes me want to cry because I can remember my parents dancing to the whole album.

Play a familiar album. Pull out a record and enjoy the whole thing. Pour a yummy drink and be transported to another place and time. Enjoy the trip.

41

Go to bed well

The best bridge between despair and hope is a good night's sleep.
—*E. Joseph Cossman*

There are nights that I feel bone weary, the kind of weary that I know will not be cured by my usual night of sleep. On those nights in particular my glowing phone and the unending loops of reels and information beckon to me in an ancient sea siren sort of way. It feels like a magnet pulling me —disguised as "rest," but I know that in order to feel truly rested, I have to do the opposite of what I feel. When I give in and rot in bed, the weariness will increase, I will stay up too late and I will find new ways to be anxious.

I figured out that the best thing I can do for myself on nights like this, is to go to bed *well*:

-Set alarm for 10 minutes of straightening my room
    -Change my sheets and make my bed, even if I'm about to get into it
    -Plug my phone far away from reach
    -Bring a book to bed, even though I usually melt into deep rest before I can read much of it.

It's simple. It's free. It's the reset my body and mind deserves.

Maybe you will make this routine your everyday gift to yourself, maybe you're like me and use it as a reset on the days you really; really need it. Either way, it's profoundly kind to set ourselves up for deep rest and renewal.

42

Sit with someone older than you.

When an old man dies, a library burns to the ground.
—*African proverb*

Something we don't get right in this postmodern age is our lack of multigenerational living. We all raise our babies in our own little houses with planned play dates run like a business arrangement. Yes, we might see our grandparents for an afternoon after church or Christmas dinner, but rarely do we experience daily living with people older than us. And because of that, we miss out on wisdom, stories, and perspective. They have lived through so many experiences; they know that the best times in life are the ones when you are furiously trying to survive, and they know that seasons of life come and go and nothing lasts forever.

SIT WITH SOMEONE OLDER THAN YOU.

There were times in my life when talking to someone much older than me felt like eating spoonfuls of hope. I was weary of only hearing from people in my own time of life, from people dealing with the same problems, doing the same routines.

Call your grandmother, go to your local park or coffee shop, and seek out someone with deep-lined wrinkles. Ask them about their life, about their loves and losses, their favorite moments, their wild stories. Not only will your perspective shift in how you view life, but you will most assuredly make someone's day by listening.

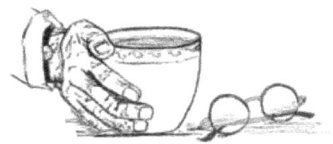

43

Look up

If we have no peace, it is because we have forgotten that we belong to each other.
—Mother Teresa

The days after my separation were consumed with chaos. I was coming out of a decade of severe depression and my world felt like it was getting smaller. I desperately wanted a break from it. One afternoon I found myself walking the streets of the little main street in my small town. Not wanting to be alone, I found a bench and sat down, coming completely into the present moment. I spent an hour just watching the people that passed by. I started off silent. I watched as lovers strolled by, their arms entwined tightly. I watched impish children wander from their parents to kick a stone. I watched an older woman in a striking purple coat inch by using her walker.

"I love that color on you!" I exclaimed not being able to stop myself. By her wide grin, I could tell I had made her day.

I waited a few more minutes and told a young woman I loved her outfit, then I made small talk with a man who sat next to me while his wife finished in a shop.

Very quickly I had forgotten all my woes. I felt connected and energized and even hopeful.

Being busy, distracted, and obsessed with our to-do lists, we don't take the time to be in our communities like we should. Just observe the travelers in an airport, everyone's neck bent as they consume through their screen—hungrily searching for connection that would be there if they just looked up.

Go plop yourself on a bench, in a coffee shop or walk a mall. But keep your head up and your smile warm. Listen to the first date, the old friends, the normal grind.

You are not alone.

44

Open all the windows

At night, I open the window
  and ask the moon to come
  and press its face against mine.
  Breathe into me.
  Close the language-door
  and open the love-window.
  The moon won't use the door,
  only the window.
  —Rumi

There's a staleness that accompanies the human experience, whether or not we are able to name why it is there; a weariness, an apathy, a boredom even. This can be called depression, a bad day, or the-kids-never-eat-their dang dinner.

OPEN ALL THE WINDOWS

If I need to be jolted out of it, I always go to my windows and throw them open. Sometimes I even open all my doors, letting the outside air come pouring into my home. 100% of the time I feel better immediately. I don't even care if it's frigidly cold outside. Even just a minute of fresh air in my home always shifts my energy.

Opening all my windows before cooking dinner is especially delicious for me. It feels like I have suddenly transported myself to a new place, even if nothing on the inside has changed. And I cook with swells of music while the new air surrounds me.

Try it. Crack your door open and stand in the gap. Let the air bathe you in newness. Throw open your windows and be transformed.

100 drops of water

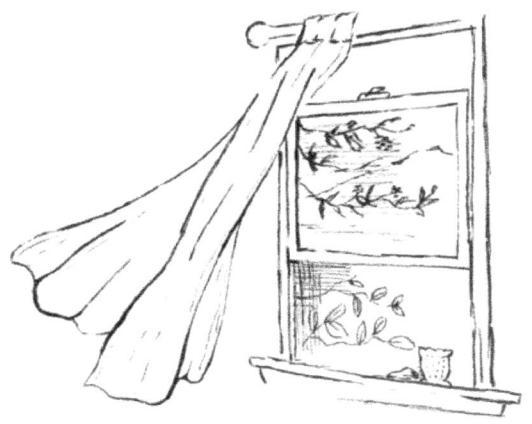

45

Bit by bit

One may walk over the highest mountain one step at a time.
　—*John Wanamaker*

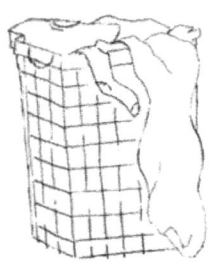

When I'm not feeling well, my house always suffers. Piles of random clutter litter places I used to enjoy and my bed is always surrounded by mountains of laundry. My brain is foggy and I wander from room to room like a lost puppy getting nothing done.

A clean home is guaranteed to make me feel a little bit better, but the process feels like Mt Everest—if Mt Everest was laundry and mail. Cleaning feels impossible. From this place of paralysis, I started something I call "bit by bit" when I was in my 30s and it has stayed with me.

One day I was in my bathroom brushing my teeth and I thought to myself…I think I could clean this room. It was a small bathroom but as I righted the things that had been upturned, wiped away the smears on the mirror, scrubbed the bathtub that had needed it for far too long…I started feeling like my brain was resting. I even ran out to the yard and plucked a few blooms from the bush near the road and put them in a little cup by the sink. It was like I was sliding into a place of putting one foot in front of the other one and it felt glorious. I got my coffee and sat on the lid of the toilet and just marveled at what it felt like to have one space that was right.

Whenever I feel like I need to slide into that place of spaciousness, I find one room and make it right.

There are many ways to do it. You can do it all by yourself if you feel strong. You can text a close friend a before picture and then an after picture. You can reward yourself for doing the task with a movie. The point is just doing a little bit.

There are some days I can't even manage to "right" a room. On these days I find myself standing in front of my jewelry drawer. I throw away earrings that don't have a mate, and arrange fun rocks that bring me joy in the space the earrings used to inhabit. It's beautiful and doable. All in all, in 5 minutes I have made order out of chaos.

Sometimes when I just feel like I am in a losing battle with stuff, I count 20 items to put away and then I reward myself. And then again and again. Hilariously I start skipping over the rewards and keep picking up things.

Bit by bit works because the house gets more peaceful; even more than that, it builds a small snowball and before I know it that productivity is propelling me to do more.

After all is said and done, my sparkling bathroom or my perfectly organized jewelry drawer shows me that I can make changes, that I am not stuck.

46

Cook something yummy

Cooking is at once child's play and adult joy. And cooking done with care is an act of love.
—Craig Claiborne

I love the act of cooking, but I cannot always get behind the tedious ingredient round-up in order to do the cooking. For a brief year it made sense for me to get a Blue Apron box in the mail and I loved that. The fun, intentional part without spending $50 on random spices a recipe called for that I would use once and store in a cabinet for decades.

What I really love is making a big thing of soup in my old yellow pot; no ingredient lists, just whatever I have on hand. I love the rhythmic motion of chopping, the way the smells start blending, even just stirring the pot slowly. It's all meditative. Add in a good playlist and it can be just plain enjoyable.

You may or may not feel like you like to cook. Cooking can be a chore when you're in a rush or when the end result is being judged. It can be a delicious treat when you take the time, when you are just enjoying the act of it. Cooking can fill your soul.

Maybe you want to spend a few hours trying out a new recipe. Maybe you want to try making bread like your grandmother used to. Maybe all you want to do is stir some sliced oranges and spices in boiling water just for the smell.

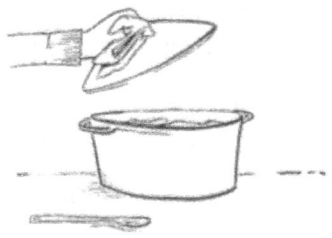

Saunter

I was out every day, and often all night, sleeping, but little, studying the so-called wonders and common things ever on show, wading, climbing, sauntering among the blessed storms and calms, rejoicing in almost everything alike that I could see or hear: the glorious brightness of frosty mornings; the sunbeams pouring over the white domes and crags into the groves end waterfalls, kindling marvelous iris fires in the hoarfrost and spray; the great forests and mountains in their deep noon sleep; the good-night alpenglow; the stars; the solemn gazing moon, drawing the huge domes and headlands one by one glowing white out of the shadows hushed and breathless like an audience in awful enthusiasm, while the meadows at their feet sparkle with frost-stars like the sky; the sublime darkness of storm-nights, when all the lights are out; the clouds in whose depths the frail snow-flowers grow; the behavior and many voices of the different kinds of storms, trees, birds, waterfalls, and snow-avalanches in the ever-changing weather.

　—John Muir

I live in an area where almost everyone hikes, in fact that is probably the number one activity that people in this area plan with their friends. The wholesomeness of hiking is attractive but deceptively for me, hiking with other people is anything but. I am trying to not breathe heavily while engaging in conversation, all the while trying to match the pace of someone with legs 30% longer than mine. I hid my distaste of hiking for years, ashamed with how much I disliked it. Then one day I learned that I love hiking by myself and even better I learned the term sauntering from reading John Muir. Because of this I no longer hike, I saunter. And by naming it, I have found others who will join me at this slow pace, focusing on wonder.

Sauntering is stopping to notice a mushroom, to go off the pathway just to see where it goes. Sauntering is stopping on a mossy patch to lay down and gaze up at the piece of sky that is framed by the tips of giant trees.

Sauntering is destination-less. It is a beautiful way to physically act out that enjoying the journey is better than the obsession with arriving somewhere. Don't get me wrong, pushing yourself to reach a summit has its own merit, but for soul comfort nothing is quite as tender to your spirit as letting yourself slowly saunter.

In a world where we are sold "wellness" at an alarming state; capitalism does not want you to know that one of the best things you can do for your brain is to put one foot in front of the other…for free. The movement of moving bilaterally does wonders for clarity, depression, and anxiety. Science proves this over and over. Walking stimulates what is used to heal PTSD patients with Eye Movement Desensitization and Reprocessing (EMDR). That movement coupled with the input of outside senses is a powerful healing tool. A good saunter will input the texture of the ferns, and the scent of fallen leaves turning to soil, the way the trunk of a tree curves, the sound of the birds calling to each other. This is the kind of input we need, especially when our phones can simultaneously bring the news of wars, death, and disease into our psyche in a matter of seconds.

When I met my husband Jimmy, I delightfully discovered that he was also a saunterer. We started what we call "bouquet walks." This is just picking up small twigs, blooms, and sticks that we find on our walk and gathering them into a little bouquet. In the winter it will be all about texture. The fluffy yellow grass, the skeleton of a leaf, the dried berries that have passed by the curiosity of the deer. In the spring the bouquet is full of every shade of beautiful color and fills two hands.

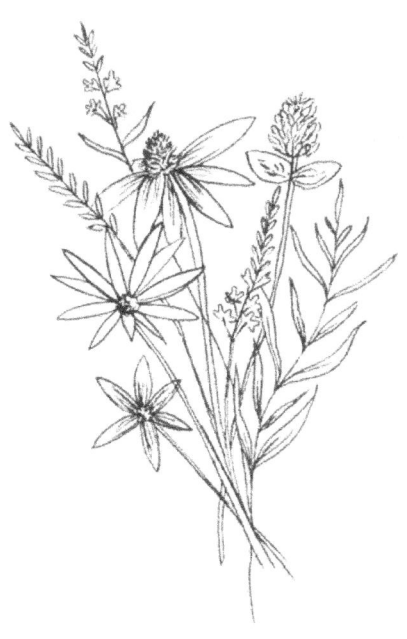

Sauntering is noticing; and noticing is some of the most powerful medicine.

Just start, one foot in front of the other.

48

Stay for dusk

Soon it got dusk, a grapy dusk, a purple dusk over tangerine groves and long melon fields; the sun the color of pressed grapes, slashed with burgundy red, the fields the color of love and Spanish mysteries.
—Jack Kerouac

I grew up on the beach and every day, right after sunset, everyone went inside to cook dinner and left me alone on the vast stretch of sand. I would run wild and barefoot, feeling like I had the whole world to myself. I found a lot of fullness in those moments because I stayed—a freedom of breath and thought. Dusk is magical to me. It feels like being wrapped in the most deliciously warm blanket.

There is something still and holy about the brief

in-between of day and night. As an adult I step outside during dusk when I want stillness or comfort. During the summer I might start to see the fireflies blinking, hear the sounds of night starting to crescendo, or catch a little piece of pink still clinging to the horizon. In the winter the bitter cold jolts me to awakeness as I wait for the stars to start shining. In the suspended space, I find that my often overactive mind is peaceful.

I always find comfort when I stay.

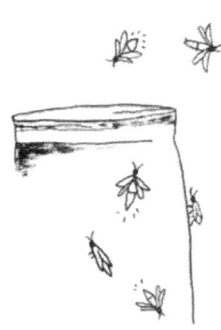

49

Visit a new town

I urge you; go find buildings and mountains and oceans to swallow you whole. They will save you, in a way nothing else can.
—*Christopher Poindexterp*

Being successful, to me, is way less about owning expensive things and more about being able to travel like I want to. After all it's what people work all their lives to do after retirement. As soul-filling as it is to hop a plane to an exotic place or a foreign city bustling with people who don't speak the same language as me, it's just not always within reach.

When I left my marriage and found myself unbearably lonely on the weekends I didn't have my children, I would start driving and find myself in a little town less than an hour away, wandering streets I'd never been to. There is something so exciting about picking a new place on the map and heading to its main street. I usually find a mix of history, art, shopping, and new foods to try all the while enjoying different architecture, parks, and people that I'm not used to seeing. Exploring reminds me that the world is so much bigger than just my little corner, even if its just a little ways down the road.

Pick a place you've never been to and explore! Go window shopping, grab a coffee, smile at someone new. Suddenly your itch to find new places isn't confined by airline miles and expensive hotels. It's just confined by your "yes".

100 drops of water

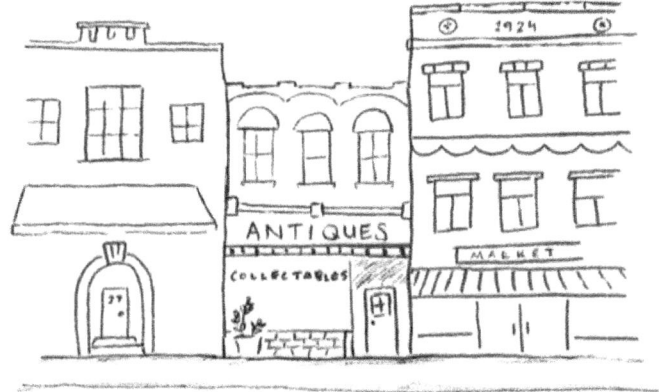

50

Sit by a fire

The most important thing in all human relationships is conversation, but people don't talk anymore, they don't sit down to talk and listen. They go to the theater, the cinema, watch television, listen to the radio, read books, but they almost never talk. If we want to change the world, we have to go back to a time when warriors would gather around a fire and tell stories.
—Paulo Coelho

Sitting around a fire was a ritual for me as a child. My great aunt Lucy would buy a bunch of hot dogs and marshmallows and host a bonfire every full moon. I remember as a child feeling so safe and comforted crouched by the flames, watching them dance around and listening to the chatter around me.

Today a simple fire brings me back to myself. The act of building the fire, tending it, and watching the flames grow and shrink is the best kind of meditation. I can glean peace from it by doing it all on my own, or if I gather friends, it brings about incredible space for stories and deep talks about life.

I can't help but think of the safety that fire brought to my ancestors. The ability to stay warm, to cook food. I can imagine generations of people with my same blood gathering around the fire, staring into it, whispering secrets and stories.

Maybe you want to meditate and build a fire all alone in the woods, enjoying the night sounds and the quiet to think. Maybe you want to host a bonfire. Maybe you have gas logs that you can turn on when you have loved ones over. Do not dismiss this simple act, taking the time to sit by a fire will bring comfort and a warmth of heart and soul.

51

Write down glimmers

Always be on the lookout for the presence of wonder.
—*E.B. White*

At the top of a quick Google search of *how to feel better*: Gratitude journaling.

In some of the depths of my seasons of depression, being told to keep a gratitude journal felt like a small adhesive bandage on a gushing wound. Laughable really.

Still, believe me, I have tried it many times.

My issue with gratitude journaling is that I KNOW what I need to be writing in it:

- I'm grateful for my family (that is falling apart).

- I'm grateful for a home (that I can barely afford)
- I'm grateful to be alive (although some days it feels impossible).

It felt like I was filling in answers to a test. It didn't feel authentic to me.

Years ago, I was having one of those days when it felt like every single thing was going wrong, I felt myself expecting things to be hard, bracing myself, and just generally feeling negative. Someone had given me a journal with wildflowers on it the day before and I pulled it out and sharpied the front "Things that have gone right"

I wrote down something so small:

I had enough milk for my cereal

Before I knew it I had filled an entire page with things that had gone right.

- *I saw a bird*
- *I could pay my light bill*
- *Someone left a quarter in the Aldi cart*

Even though these were technically things I was

grateful for, it almost took it to a more cellular level. The simplest of discoveries. I found there was incredible power in shifting my mindset from feeling like nothing is going right to noticing glimmers of beauty and hope.

I do not do this every day, only when things feel really hard. Years later, I heard that what I was writing down were also known as "glimmers."

100 drops of water

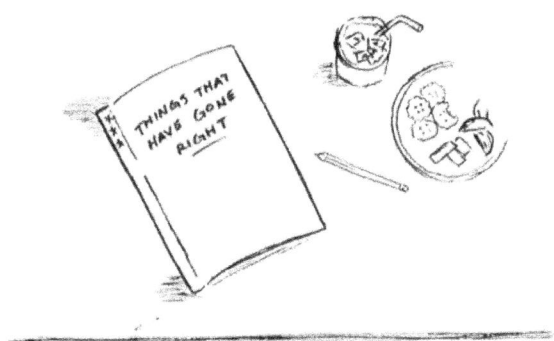

Maybe you want to designate a beautiful journal for this practice. Maybe you want to do it every single day. Maybe you want to scratch it out on an old receipt and call it a day. Maybe you want to share with friends, or start a group where you share glimmers with others. All it really takes is noticing.

52

Cry

There is a sacredness in tears. They are not the mark of weakness, but of power.
—Washington Irving

I have long been a champion of a cleansing cry for quite some time. Sometimes nothing else will do. The physical experience of not holding back grief or frustration is transformative and moves it through my body in a way that helps me move forward.

How to cry:

- tell yourself it's ok
- sit with the uncomfortable silence of just being

How to cry faster:

- music
- photos
- visiting a place that reminds you of something or someone
- driving
- being alone
- practice crying. . .it will get easier

53

Make room

The question of what you want to own is actually the question of how you want to live your life.
—*Marie Kondō*

Right after a year of mental health issues that pretty much debilitated me, I found myself in a home with piles and piles of stuff around me–stuff that hadn't been dealt with and had been pushed to the side. It was the same home I had the year before, yet I felt like a stranger in it. I wanted to move on with my life, to truly start living in the present instead of the past —only my home felt like a prison.

That was the year that Marie Kondō came out with the delightful little book *The Life Changing Magic of Tidying Up*. You might even have it stashed on a book shelf right now of "read some day" books. That little book gave me a road map to getting my house back in order. I remember piling every piece of clothing I owned in the living room and carefully going through each piece to see what sparked joy. I found myself donating dresses that would never fit me, sweaters that were too itchy, an outfit that reminded me of a really bad day. And when I put what remained back in my closet it felt so joyful! I purged every closet and every drawer in the house over the next few months. I became obsessed with making even my sock drawer a place that felt good and peaceful. She was right! It was life-changing.

Now, most people don't have the luxury of the time, or even the energy that is needed to organize a home that way. But even on a very small scale, taking an hour or a day or a week to really purge what is no longer serving you, will allow for more beautiful present moments to take place in your space.

Maybe this book, translated from Japanese, seems silly and over the top but you can take the basic bones of the whole thing and apply it to whatever you want. And the basic bones are this:

Don't keep things you aren't using or don't love.

Making room, making peace, and letting go of things that no longer serve you are wonderful habits to lean into. And they have wonderful end results. Making room for more beauty and life is always a good thing.

- Choose one place. (I would suggest your closet or your bedroom.)
- Create keep, donate, or throw away piles.
- Let the process unfold with no judgment and lots of curiosity.
- Enjoy

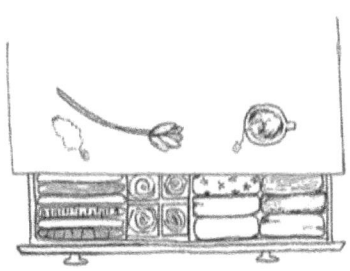

54

Get cozy

O for a life of sensations rather than of thoughts.
—*John Keats*

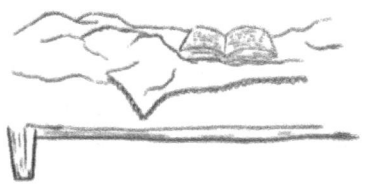

If you haven't heard of the Danish art of hygge (pronounced hoo-ga) I highly recommend looking into it. There are several books out right now that are equally lovely in explaining this approach to living. A way of living that is far outside of the way we live here in the US. Objectively it's because it cultivates satisfaction with what we *have* instead of what capitalism tells us we need—preying on our insecurities.

Hygge is the art of coziness that has been cultivated from the long Danish winters. Hygge is about bringing light into our dark homes with fire or candles, leaning into softness, tea, simple decor, and warm wooly socks. It is making a nest in your home that holds you.

I've found even in the other three seasons that practicing hygge when I am needing some soul nourishment feels wonderful and takes minimal effort.

Being cozy could/should be a normal thing that every single person can achieve no matter how much money they have. You don't need access to expensive home good stores or tons of time to set up spaces of coziness, you just need to work with what you've got.

Maybe as you lean into this Danish art, you embrace it and transform your home bit by bit to a hygge sanctuary. Maybe you make a little corner of your house a space for you to just sink into and rest, a reading nook, a "drink tea and watch the birds space." Maybe try it for one evening with whatever you can scrape together (which will be more than you think).

3 steps for making something hygge:

- clear a space of clutter (this can be a single chair all the way to a whole room)
- light a candle
- wrap something soft around you
- indulge yourself with softness and rest

55

Have a guilt free lazy day

You gotta know when to be lazy. Done correctly, it's an art form that benefits everyone.
—*Nicholas Sparks*

In the midst of the busy summers when my babies were little, I would find myself in August as threadbare as one can be. No amount of sleep could revive me out of what felt like an eternal exhaustion. That combined with the heat and the long days brought me to a point of one day saying, "I need to go to a hotel for a night." One brief night. Just me.

I found one on a weekday for not a lot of money and packed to go. I spent the next 18 hours taking baths, sleeping sprawled out and naked on the crisp white sheets. I ordered take out, binge watched

Project Runway on my computer, and did absolutely no self-evaluation, no organizing, no goal planning and best of all, no guilt.

The key was deciding to have the day, being intentional. Because doing all of those things on days I needed to be productive would spiral me into feeling worse about myself.

Now my kids are older and I have more time to myself. But I still value the intentionality of a guilt free lazy day.

Humans need rest. We need pre-adulting kind of languishing time. We need to lose ourselves in a show or a book, eat what sounds good, and engage in a "not be bothered" kind of rest.

You don't have to book a hotel for it (although it is quite nice if it's in your budget). But setting an intentional day of divine nothingness can make a huge difference.

Doing nothing every once in a while is a gift to yourself.

100 drops of water

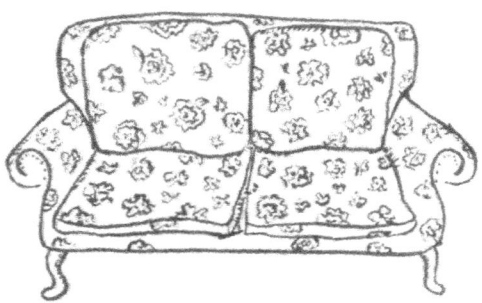

56

Gaze at the stars

If people looked at the stars each night, they'd live a lot differently.
—Bill Watterson

Something I love about stars is that the darker it is, the more brilliant they shine. And just the same, the deeper I am in depression, the more life changing it is to take a moment to look up and see the night sky.

All at once I am both small and meaningful. My place here on earth is surely so purposeful and so important.

It is free to have a front row seat to the wonders of the galaxies. Sometimes as I unload my car after a long day, I will stand, leaned against my porch steps, in awe that on an ordinary day, the sky can be that magnificent. Sometimes it is the promise of a blood moon, or a meteor shower that gets me to stop what I'm doing, grab a blanket to lay on, and go watch the sky.

Whether it's for a few moments after you put your kids to bed, on a blanket with someone you love, or sitting by a campfire in a giant open place, don't forget to look at the stars.

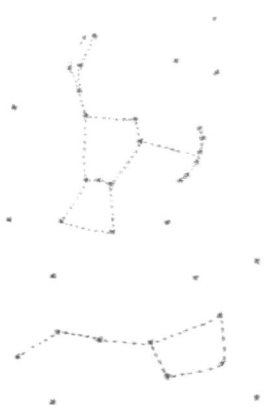

57

Make a self portrait

I paint self-portraits because I am so often alone, because I am the person I know best.
—Frida Kahlo

The art of the self-portrait is ages old, dating way before iPhone selfies have taken over the internet. In a culture where vanity and self-centeredness is rampant, why take the time to do a self portrait?

Because taking the time to *slow down* and sit with yourself for a while is healing, no matter what stage or phase you are in.

If you are angry, taking the time to sit with yourself, to feel the anger, and to try to capture it will in the end help you process through the anger.

If you are sad, take that time to lean into your sadness.

If you feel messy, tired, overwhelmed, or hopeful—finding a way to convey that in a photograph of yourself is a way to deal with the feelings head on.

I find it a way of marking seasons of my life. A little ritual when I know I need to move on.

I first stumbled onto self portraits when I was 12 years old with my mother's old film camera. I would set up dramatic scenes, pose, and have my little sisters snap the shutter. It wasn't even about the end result as much as it was about setting it up, deciding what lighting, what setting, how to arrange my body and limbs–the emotion I wanted to convey in my eyes.

I have continued my self portrait journey throughout highs and lows of my life. New motherhood, depression, mania, divorce, and just the human experience.

I have propped up my phone in a pile of laundry, shot my eye wrinkles in my mirror, and captured my reflection in water. I wouldn't use "pretty" to describe the results. Instead…haunting, moving, stirring. There's a lot of freedom in making something that isn't pretty, that isn't for other people's approval.

MAKE A SELF PORTRAIT

Take a self-portrait of where you are right now. Give yourself one shot. Don't overthink it.

Edit it in black and white (one of my favorite tricks for making normal photos more moody).

Photograph yourself through a journey. The beginning and the middle and the end.

Photograph yourself for a set number of days. 7, 30, 100.

Show up, sit with yourself and see what you see, you might be surprised how much you like it.

58

Go to the ocean

We have salt in our blood, in our sweat, in our tears. We are tied to the ocean.
　—*John F Kennedy*

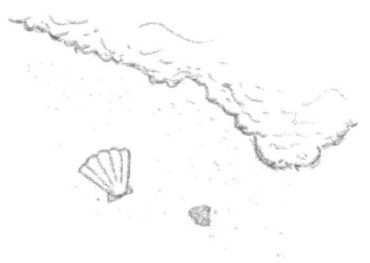

Some of my clearest thinking has happened with my toes in the Atlantic or Pacific ocean and my gaze to the horizon. I always say it makes me feel so small and yet so important. The endless gaze of the horizon, the vastness of the ocean—it is both a holy and a healing place to be. In a way, I think that all humans feel belonging there at the edge of it all.

I sometimes imagine looking at the earth from outer space and seeing the edges of the land lined with people looking *out*. People connecting in *that feeling* no matter where their location is on the planet.

For me, the magic of the ocean is not as much in being in the water (I do have a fear of what lurks in the murky salt waters I grew up around). But the magic is in standing on the edge of something that is endless, and yet feeling the steady lap of the waves on my toes and the certain rising and falling of tides.

Get to the ocean, if even for a day. Sit on the edge, wrap yourself in a blanket if it's cold, behold the majesty of it.

Watch some comedy

Always laugh when you can, it is cheap medicine.
 —*Lord Byron*

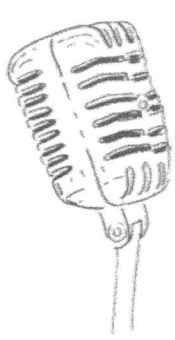

WATCH SOME COMEDY

After my divorce, I found myself feeling so alone on Monday nights. Lonely and lost. All of my community and friends were busy with their kiddos, doing homework and doing dishes. One profound night, I found myself at a seedy bar with a comedy open mic night. The hours that followed were filled with laughter until I cried. The kind that feels SO DAMN good. Sometimes, I didn't even think something was funny, like the guy who told the same sandwich joke every single week for 6 months, and that just made me laugh harder.

Mondays became my favorite day as I would show up, get two Shirley Temples at the bar, and find myself lost in laughter for the next three hours. Laughing like that was life changing. It felt like the rattling in my body literally shook depression out of me.

Comedy can be shocking and crass but there are many clean comics or comedy clubs. For me, some of the beauty of the shocking kind of comedy is a peek into the human mind. I started saying that going to comedy was like going to the modern art museum of brains.

Find an open mic night in your area, buy a ticket to a comedy show, listen to a stand up on Netflix. Just get to laughing as soon as you can.

And do it often.

60

Say what you feel

Just be honest with yourself. That opens the door.
—*Vernon Howard*

All the best changes in my life happened because I got honest about how I felt. One of my biggest core values is honesty and yet I am a master at making things more beautiful than they are, romanticizing shitty things, and pretending I'm ok when I'm not. I'm honest to other people and not always with myself.

Once in a while, I challenge myself to a "saying how I really feel day."

It feels silly, it feels like it would be in the same category as a comedic "say yes day" movie.

It starts right away when the first stranger says

"Hey how's it going?" and I bite my tongue from saying "fine"

I might reply, "You know, I'm feeling really achey today." I don't trauma dump, and I don't just say "bad," but I challenge myself to a moment of truth.

It doesn't always happen right away, but replying in this way opens things up to more connection, more conversation, and even if no one knows what to say, you've said your truth and that in itself is day changing.

Do it for a grocery shopping trip, do it for an hour, do a whole day if you're feeling adventurous. You will truly not believe how differently you will feel at the end of the day having taken off your mask and having said what you really feel.

61

Give yourself a sound track

Tell me what you listen to, and I'll tell you who you are.
—*Tiffanie DeBartolo*

I had an aunt who would clean her kitchen with the soundtrack to Gladiator blasting through the speakers. That's right. My little, conservative aunt would put in her Gladiator CD and suddenly she was in her own world conquering, cleaning or cooking with all the intensity that Hans Zimmer could compose.

I have found that turning on music can change everything. It can motivate me, it can shift my mood, it can help me get lost in whatever task I am doing. Suddenly simple actions, accompanied by cinematic swells, are more enjoyable.

When I'm sad and need to cry, I listen to coal mining ballads. When I need to clean, I put on rap songs from my college clubbing days. When I want to get lost in cooking I put on Vivaldi's Four Seasons.

Experiment with different soundtracks for your life. See how it feels to romanticize even the most mundane moments.

We have to live life, including all the ups and downs, we might as well have beautiful music to accompany us.

62

Write about a memory

Tell me a fact, and I'll learn. Tell me a truth, and I'll believe. But tell me a story, and it will live in my heart forever.
   —*Ed Sabol*

100 drops of water

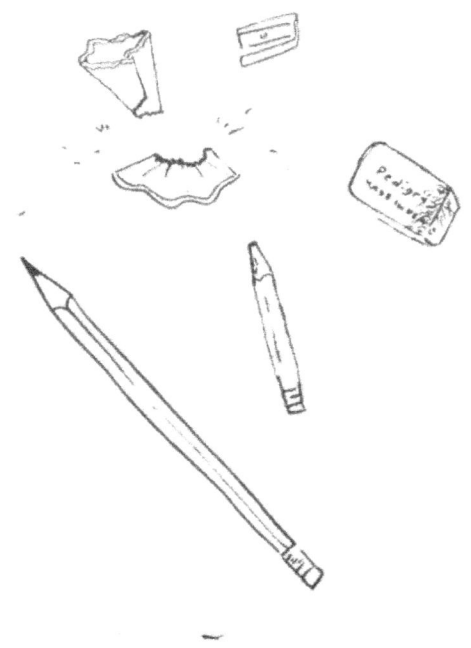

WRITE ABOUT A MEMORY

I went to a writing workshop once and was given the task of writing out one of my favorite memories. Simple enough. I was expecting something more deep, more thought provoking or difficult. As soon as I started, my body changed. I was suddenly IN the story. My pen flew over paper because this memory had so much to it: the smells, the feel of the ocean on my ankles, the way the rain pelted my pregnant belly. It all came out with a steady flow and choosing the words to tell it was incredibly delightful. It was a full submersive experience.

Writing is overwhelming to a lot of people. We want to get it right, we want to say things just so, but so much of the joy of writing is just doing it. And telling a story that you treasure is a great way to do it.

Not only will it have you reliving a nice memory, but it will help you remember it in a lot of new ways.

Maybe you never show your memory story to a single soul and just experience the joy of writing it. Maybe you share it with a family member, or pass it to your children, or mail it to your friend.

Let yourself get lost in story telling—in describing how something felt, tasted, looked, sounded, and looked. There is no wrong way.

63

Make a space lovely with what you've got

The power of finding beauty in the humblest things makes home happy and life lovely.
—Louisa May Alcott

Decorating a space can make it go from a place you avoid to a place that feels homey and nice. Decorating also, to some people, sounds like a huge headache and a huge expense. And it can be.

Sometimes when I just need a little umph to my week, I will spruce up a space and change things around. Did you ever do that as a kid? Way before iPads and the internet, I would rearrange my room every few weeks. I would shift the bed and the dresser and mix things up so it felt new.

I still do the same things sometimes and "shop my

house" for ways to spruce it up. I also usually go outside and use elements from nature to help make it special.

This might look like tying colored leaves to an old hoop I used to cross stitch with and making a little mobile, or just a handful of flowers in a glass jar.

I will shift and sort and trade out art until it feels new.

The key to this is not falling into the trap of having to go to the store to get new stuff. You don't need new stuff, you just need to get back to that childhood joy of working with what you have.

100 drops of water

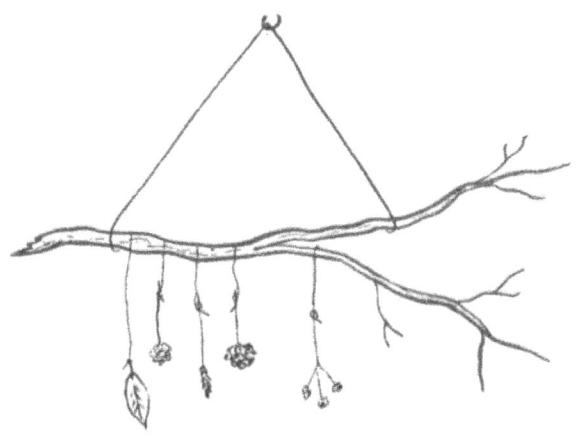

64

Try it sober

When I got sober, I thought giving up was saying goodbye to all the fun and all the sparkle, and it turned out to be just the opposite. That's when the sparkle started for me.
—Mary Karr

Sobriety is a nuanced word. Some people do medicate themselves with the classic vices of alcohol or drugs. But that isn't the only thing that we numb ourselves with. We numb ourselves with social media, scrolling. . .and even with healthy things like podcasts or food. Numb is a state in which we don't have to feel as deeply or connect with others in a normal way. And living like this constantly keeps us from beauty and connection!

I am convinced that more than half the world is walking around numb and disconnected.

Being present can feel AWFUL, itchy, and uncomfortable. And sometimes we can't stay awake for long before slipping back to numbness. For me social media is this black hole that is constantly calling to me. I can be in a space that is full of connection and I will find my thumb longing to scroll my phone in that numbing dance I always do. For a friend of mine it's drinking half a bottle of wine at night. Neither is worse, both are keeping us from our best existence.

Maybe you want to get sober from something. Like all the way, "AA meetings and chips" type of sober. Maybe you need to challenge yourself to hours or minutes with your phone shut off, or an evening where you choose to forgo the bottle of wine and instead sit on the porch and listen to the birds winding down.

Play with it. Look at periods of sobriety as a gift instead of a chore. Give yourself gifts when you can. I promise that your senses will be filled and your heart will be changed in the process…no matter how long you do it for.

65

Read a good book

You think your pain and your heartbreak are unprecedented in the history of the world, but then you read. It was books that taught me that the things that tormented me most were the very things that connected me with all the people who were alive, who had ever been alive.
—*James Baldwin*

Getting lost in a book is a luxury. Even though picking up a book doesn't take a lot of money or effort, I still find myself scrolling on my phone when I used to read. Reading a good book feels like eating a healthy meal after traveling for a week and only eating junk food. Reading is a kindness to yourself in so many ways, a big pile of veggies for your brain.

Once in a while I will read a novel or get sucked

into a series. What I really treat myself with is poetry. Slipping into my bath with a new poetry book feels like the best way to fill my soul back up. It takes me out of my own consciousness, my own thinking and overanalyzing. There is a space, a quieting of external factors, and a deep connecting to *others*.

If I'm on a trip I usually will try to get into a fiction book. I remember devouring Hunger Games on the beach in the Caribbean and the luxury of just lounging for hours, lost in a world my mind had created. Sometimes I forget that reading can happen any time.

Maybe you want to try something simple to stretch those muscles of presence by reading a book of poetry—even if you "don't get it." Maybe you want to add a ritual of reading before bed every night. Maybe you want to research what the cool kids are into these days and try it out. Maybe you want to download an audiobook and listen to it while you're doing the after school grind.

Give reading a chance. Give it time to sink into your bones, to take over your mind, to give you more insight into other cultures and ways of life. There is literally no place you cannot go.

READ A GOOD BOOK

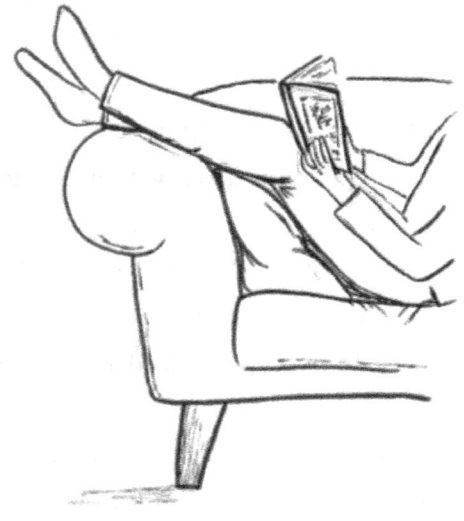

66

Arrange flowers

Happiness is the art of making a bouquet of those flowers within reach.
—*Bob Goddard*

Picking flowers is such a beautiful activity, but arranging them can be just as fun. I think of it as painting with blooms. It's important to remind yourself that there is no "right way" to arrange flowers. Some people love symmetry and cohesion, some people love simple designs—like the modern Japanese style, Ikebana. Then there are people like me who love arranging the wildest, most abstract bouquet of flowers with little to no plan.

Things that make flower arranging fun for me:

- a metal floral frog makes arranging flowers stay better
- finding things with texture that are NOT flowers. This could be grass, a cool stick, a feather, or a vine.
- having some short and some long stems
- making one side a little higher so it sort of *swoops* the eye
- taking leaves off of some stems so it's not so crowded

Once you start, you'll get more confident, more excited, and more eager. It's now a treat for myself to forage my yard, grab a few blooms from Trader Joes', and have an arrangement that can bring me joy for a week.

But again and again, it's the process that's the magic—not necessarily the end result.

Try your hand at arranging some flowers, see what you end up creating!

67

Be with different generations

A generation is like a book, they all have a theme and a lesson to be learned.
—*William Saroyan*

Nothing can put things into perspective like being with people that aren't your age. I love being around people older and younger than me and being inspired by their wisdom and their wonder. We have gradually drifted from situations like this in our families and in our communities but I'm here to say we NEED to bring this back. Everyone needs everyone…in fact, someone needs YOU. That's right. There is someone in your community who would absolutely benefit from being in a relationship with you. Maybe it's an elderly person who feels like their lives are over, who might be inspired to hear what you're doing or dealing with. . .and hey! they might even have some wisdom to share. Or maybe there's a kid who needs someone to look up to, someone to see them and tell them they're doing a great job.

We can listen to each other's stories, make sure everyone is getting their needs met, and provide encouragement and connection for people outside of our generation.

Find places for this: community spaces, community picnics, volunteer for a festival, host a family reunion, go to your local coffee shop and strike up a conversation.

68

Nourish yourself

That's something I've noticed about food: whenever there's a crisis if you can get people to eating normally, things get better.
—*Madeleine L'Engle*

When I get depressed, I always forget the basics: food, water, taking a shower, getting dressed, getting good sleep. In fact, when I am not doing well, I tend to sabotage myself by doing the exact opposite of what I need.

I can't tell you how many times complete and total meltdowns were avoided just by eating something.

When I feel stuck, sometimes I have to think

about the opposite of what I want to do and do that: treat myself like I am a little child:

Feed myself something nourishing, get in the shower, go outside in the sun, put my phone away, and say "no" to that last Netflix show and get some sleep.

I think the key is viewing ourselves as valuable and important enough to provide these necessities.

Something I have to remind myself of daily if I'm feeling bad:

Have you eaten something healthy?
Have you taken a shower?
Have you drunk water recently?
Have you been outside?
Have you gotten enough sleep?
Have you talked with a friend?

If the answer is no, you've got some work to do. Not only do you deserve having your needs met, but you will find that meeting your needs allows you to actually have a better chance at enjoying life.

69

Write yourself a letter

Your vision will become clear only when you can look into your own heart. Who looks outside, dreams; who looks inside, awakes.
—*Carl Jung*

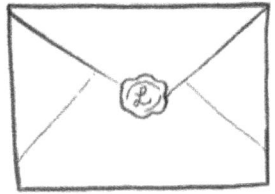

There are lots of ways to inwardly reflect. There's journaling, therapy, meditation, and other things like writing prompts. I love all of them. As I have grown, healed, and changed, I have found myself thinking of myself as having just become a new version of myself. I like thinking this way because it feels accurate—*I am always becoming.*

Something I love doing to keep track of the different changes is writing letters to myself.

It started one Christmas evening. Everyone was playing with new toys or napping on the couch and I was taking down the tree in an effort to keep pine needles from sticking to the bottom of my feet everywhere I went, and also to regain a sense of simplicity again. That evening I was thinking of the season like I usually did. Things that went wrong, things that went right. And I realized that it seemed like I had the same sort of thoughts every Christmas:

Why did I drink so much damn eggnog?

Why do I never have food in the fridge on Christmas eve?

Why do I fall into the lie that kids need MORE activities when they really don't like being run all around town?

That night I wrote a letter to myself and stuck it in the top of the Christmas box of ornaments. The following Christmas I was surprised to see it sitting there at the top and I had forgotten even writing it. That Christmas was different as I kept some things in mind. It has now been 10 years of this ritual and I love the tradition. I look forward to seeing the growth, the changes, the love. I love being reminded that we will not stay the same. Some years are humorous and lighthearted, some years are riddled with pain…and yet I always made it through.

I like to do this with the new year, new seasons, childrens' birthdays, important milestones. Just a little letter to myself to check in and say "hey! you're doing it."

Maybe you do it once and tuck it somewhere to find one day, maybe you want to create a ritual that you can follow so that you are doing it more.

What would your letter say?

70

Dare to dream

Nothing happens unless first we dream.
　—*Carl Sandburg*

Manifesting is really sexy right now and I have to say. . .I'm into it. Maybe the word itself feels a bit contrived, but the call to dream and dream intentionally feels magical and right. It reminds me of my girlhood when I would tear things out of magazines and glue them together in a patchwork quilt of desires. It feels delicious to be that hopeful girl again, even in my 40s.

Because the older I get, the more I really feel the possibility of things. I know people in their 70s absolutely killing it with living their most treasured lives. It is never too late to reroute!

Daring to dream about how things could be, and dreaming in a way that is so alive with detail actually helps magnetize making it happen. I have seen it over and over again. If we don't dream, if we don't name what it is we want, I can promise you that you will not just stumble on it.

A way that you could dream out loud:

- Pick 10 things (places you want to go, how you want to FEEL, how you want to spend your days, an outfit you want to wear, even something you want to own)
- Look up art, photos, or create digital words or art
- Screenshot it
- Print photos from your phone
- Tape them on a wall that you see every day
- Take them in, feel the reality of them, and see what happens
- Don't be afraid to dream

71

Give a compliment

A compliment is something like a kiss through a veil.
—*Victor Hugo*

I love giving genuine compliments. I do it quite often and that's mostly because the reaction I get is intoxicating, a little burst of joy.

"Oh my goodness you look beautiful in that shade of blue!"

"Sir, can I just say, that is the coolest tattoo I've ever seen!"

"Wow! I love your tutu! Does it twirl?" (said to a little toddler at the grocery store)

It doesn't have to be complicated or long but taking the time to compliment someone (even a stranger) will cheer up two people.

Try giving 5 genuine compliments today. This is an act of noticing, of looking for the good, of being on the look out for beauty and saying so!

Go camping

Wilderness is not a luxury, but a necessity of human spirit.
—*Edward Abbey*

Oh camping—the absolute bane of my existence and something that actually holds so many of my favorite memories.

Camping takes so much prep and so much recovery. I don't ever sleep well, on the first night at least; it's dirty, and the ground hurts my hips, and if you told someone in a third world country that we leave our comfy homes to sleep on the ground in a tent they would think you were mad. But camping ALWAYS brings me to a place of wildness that I need. Something about cooking over a fire, sitting under the stars, going to bed with a river in my ear…

it pricks at a primal part of who I am. It must do a lot for other people since camping is a huge industry and honestly, at times, a sign of privilege that people "get to go camping."

Here's the thing. You do not have to go all in to get the benefits of camping. If full on tent camping isn't your thing, here's some ways to make it more accessible.

- Sleep outside. You can pull your mattress onto a porch, sleep in a hammock, rent one of those glamping tents with a full on bed in them
- Cook outside. Sometimes when I don't have it in me to do a whole trip, I will take hotdogs and s'mores and build a fire by the river and then return to my comfy bed for the night
- Make a fire and sit around it
- Go hiking
- Get out in nature and remind yourself you're a wild little soul.

GO CAMPING

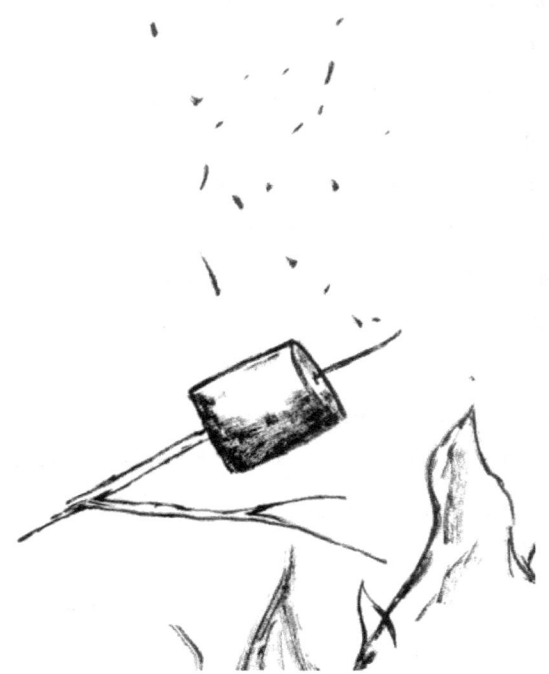

73

Climb to the top

The summit is what drives us, but the climb itself is what matters.
—*Conrad Anker*

One of the darkest periods of time in my life was the year before I left my marriage. The year I woke up to the truth of how unhappy I was. This year was muddy, hard, and I felt paralyzed.

There is a mountain near my house that people climb for fun. And by climbing I mean walking straight up for a mile and a half to an overlook, not anything that involves a harness and carabiners. I had done it a few times in my life and I hated every minute of it. That December I decided as an act of faith in myself that I was going to climb it 52 times (once a week) in 2020. Spoiler alert, I did it. Spoiler alert, I still hate it BUT I learned so much about myself while showing up 52 times to do it.

I documented my climbs that year and the lessons I learned. I started doing it with friends and documenting our conversations and the things I learned from them. Mostly though, it was the constant reminder that one foot in front of the other would eventually get you somewhere. As simple as that is, it was hard to remember. After that year of climbing, I saw my life dramatically change as I put one foot in front of the other in other areas of my life.

Maybe you aren't athletic and climbing a mountain feels impossible. Go climb a hill, take the stairs to the top of the tall building near you, run to the top of the bleachers at the local baseball stadium.

The crazy thing is you can actually do it. You can do it as slowly as a sloth, but if you keep putting one foot in front of the other you will get there eventually.

Climb something and be ready to change.

74

Pick something

Right now I just want to chill for a while. Take a hiatus from all the craziness. To clean my house, see my family. Just see some movies and pick some strawberries.

—*Lauren Ambrose*

PICK SOMETHING

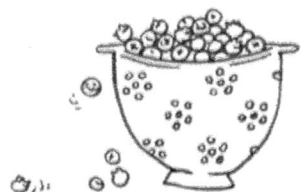

I've always thought it was so funny that orchards or farms offer *picking* for more than it would cost to just buy their fruits or vegetables. That tells you something. That the act of harvesting food is so enjoyable that they can actually charge people to do the work for them.

Our ancestors used to be way more involved in the process of getting food on the table. Maybe they had a garden or worked in one. The work was rewarding in many ways.

I remember going strawberry picking as a little girl. I would pick two and eat one and end the day with sticky hands and a full belly. I loved the search for just the right ripeness, the sound it made when I plucked it off the vine, and the satisfaction of a basket full of berries to bring home.

I live in a place where apple orchards surround our town like a little frame. Every fall I take my kids to pick apples EVEN THOUGH a bag of apples from the grocery story down the road is 1/8th the price. The experience is just so fun it brings us back every year.

Go pick something. Harvest your garden, pick out a pumpkin, gather berries or apples or lemons. Get back to that feeling of ancient wonder that our food grows from the ground and that it is DELICIOUS.

Put your phone down

The moment is not found by seeking it, but by ceasing to escape from it.
—*James Pierce*

I am 100% convinced that a big contributor to the undercurrent of dissatisfaction in our lives is that we have access to everything at all times in our hand held phones. Never has a society had so much power and yet it is the undoing of so much of life's simple pleasures.

Did you know that you are being advertised to almost every moment of your day unless you have gone to great lengths to shut down apps, or get a dumb phone? Have you checked your screen time recently? Or counted how many times your thumb goes to scroll in a 5 minute period when you feel bored? It's a lot for the average human.

Putting down your phone is hard. We do so much on it; it makes us feel productive and powerful and sometimes connected and yet the setting down of that power can open us up to living life as it was meant to be—in the present, with our senses fully engaged.

Look out the window, be bored, let your imagination go. Play with your kids, go for a walk, talk to someone with all of your attention.

These things that used to be normal are life giving.

Maybe you can only give up an hour today. Set a timer. It will feel uncomfortable at first but see where it takes you. Maybe you want to go a whole day with it shoved in a drawer. Maybe you want to challenge yourself to shutting it off after dinner or starting your mornings without turning it on.

Give your brain a break and see what unfolds.

76

Go for a drive

Sometimes you find yourself in the middle of nowhere and sometimes in the middle of nowhere you find yourself.
—Stacy Westfall

With gas prices as high as they are, driving with no purpose is not as popular as it once was. However, once in a while, taking a drive to nowhere is exactly what the soul needs. Turn on some music, open your windows, stick your hand outside and let it float on the wind like you did when you were a child. Turn down that windy road you pass every day on the way to work. The one you've always wondered about. Get off at an exit you've never been on. Sing at the top of your lungs because you don't have an audience. Cry too if that's what you need. Let the mindless experience of taking a sacred drive meet you where you are. You don't have to be anything, do anything, arrive anywhere.

You just need to be held and the road can do that.

77

Sit in the sun

The sun does not shine for a few trees and flowers, but for the wide world's joy.
—*Henry Ward Beecher*

If I feel blah, nothing wakes me up like the sun.

Besides the scientific properties of getting more vitamin D which has a lot to do with our mood, sitting in the sun is an undeniable spiritual experience. I always sit crosslegged on the earth and lift my face to the sun with my eyes gently closed. I love how it feels to have that brightness right there behind my eyelids—brightness so big I can't even look at it. I love the sensation of how it feels on my face and pours over my body like warm syrup. Just five minutes can absolutely shake me out of a funk.

Maybe it's winter and you want to travel to a place where you can be in the sun a lot. Maybe you drag yourself outside and let the sun wake you up just a little during your lunch break. Maybe you work outside for a few hours or take a walk in the park on a sunny day.

Let the sun remind you that you are alive. Let it warm you from your inside out.

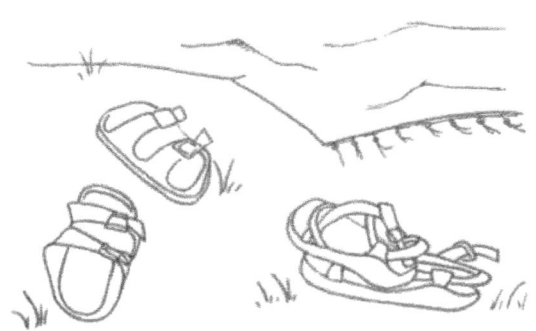

Meditate

In awareness there is no becoming, there is no end to be gained. There is silent observation without choice and condemnation, from which there comes understanding.
—*Jiddu Krishnamurti*

I am not who you think of when you imagine the kind of person who meditates. I don't talk softly, I am not quiet, and I sure as hell have too many thoughts to even pretend to be peaceful. I wrote it off for many years as "not my thing".

And then I saw a little video describing what meditation really is, which is not emptying your mind of thoughts, but simply letting the thoughts come and go until you come to a place of presence. The key to all of this was the big kicker—you don't judge the thoughts.

I tried it, thinking I would surely fail. And very, very quickly I realized that you can't fail something you aren't judging. Each time I mediated, I found it easier to just be like "yep. . .moving on"

I also learned I was already meditating when I floated in the ocean on my back, or when I laid in bed at night. When I let my thoughts flow.

For me, meditation became a tool for me to get back to BEING and stop with the churning and doing.

Myths of meditation:

- That it needs to be quiet—you can meditate in the middle of a busy street
- That you need to be sitting in cross legged position (I meditate best on my back with my legs and arms sprawled out)
- That only hippy-dippy granola people meditate
- That it is religious
- That you can do it wrong

Start off small, do a Youtube meditation, look up

community resources, or give yourself 10 minutes during your lunch break to simply see what happens.

79

Do something you're good at

Success is liking yourself, liking what you do and liking how you do it.
—Maya Angelou

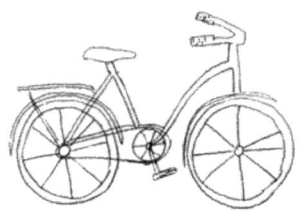

DO SOMETHING YOU'RE GOOD AT

When I feel apathetic about life, I have a little trick that always works to bring me back to a state of wanting to actively participate in mine. And it is simply to do something I'm good at. This could be an extension of my job as a photographer, where I photograph someone for a project or at a new location to test it out. At first it may seem awkward and weird but the second I slide behind my lens, something takes over. I am suddenly doing something I have honed over the years and doing it well. I am flooded with pleasure as I keep on. Sometimes it's doing something like writing a poem that's been living in me. And sometimes it is something mostly physical like dancing.

Maybe for you it is a craft you used to enjoy and that you excel at-- something that you don't make time for anymore. Maybe it's going for a run to remind you that you are strong. Maybe you need to volunteer for something that comes easy to you, where your skills can bless people who need it.

Even if you don't do the thing for long, stepping into those places of being excellent at something is a powerful way to revive your soul.

Everyone is good at something. Dust off your crafts, challenge your body to remember its muscle memory, and do what you've worked hard to be good at.

80

Wear clothes that fit

A woman is never sexier than when she is comfortable in her own clothes.
—*Vera Wang*

Screw sizing. I hate it. I can be a size 12 in one brand and a 20 in another. Not only does this mess with my mind but it makes me wear things that don't fit just based on the little number on the tag. Human bodies change and they really change during dark times. Some people lose weight and some people gain weight. I am the latter in that statement. But I tell you what doesn't make me feel better if I've gained weight and that is forcing myself to wear something that presses in on my stomach or makes me feel like it is pulling on me. I don't like wearing things that I have to be posed *just so* for it to look ok. I want to be living and walking through the world NOT thinking about how I look in something.

Wearing clothes that fit is a game changer. It's hard to put away things you WISH you could wear but it's way better to wear clothes that fit the body you have—even if you're planning on pulling out your old clothes again one day.

Go shopping (I shop at thrift stores—which is great for my budget and my often changing body). Start with one outfit that fits you perfectly that allows you to go through your day comfortably. Perks if they are in colors or patterns that you love, as you don't have to wear all black to look your best. Cut the tags out of them if the number bothers you and enjoy how it feels to harvest all of that energy that has been being siphoned from your life because you have felt awkward in the clothes you wear.

You will see how much better you feel.

81

Call a friend

No friendship is an accident.
—O. Henry

In my lifetime (I'm nearly 40), I have seen such an incredible shift in how we interact with our friends. And it's not good. When I was a child, I would sit on my sunporch, on top of the black and pink chaise lounge and talk to my friend Kathrine for hours. I would loop the curly chord of the cream colored phone around my fingers, and get lost in our conversation. I don't remember much of what we talked about, but I remember how it felt to have a friend on the other end of the line.

Nowadays I rarely ever get a phone call, instead

I'm pinged with countless texts that overwhelm me and keep my phone glowing.

I don't know why but it has gotten to the point where a phone call means that something bad has happened. We plan phone calls like we used to plan outings, and still, it feels awkward.

Yet, a long conversation with a friend is like the greatest healing elixir, or the biggest inhale of fresh air. For a long season of life, I was driving for an hour late at night and ended up reconnecting with a friend on the West coast. I had a little ritual of chatting about my week with her. It wasn't anything huge but it was something I looked forward to every week.

So pick up your phone and call a friend. Maybe even text a quick "Nothing is wrong, just wanted to hear your voice" text before you do. Maybe you'll like that so much you'll make a habit of connecting with someone weekly so it becomes more natural and expected.

We were made to need our friends and I'm sorry but texts are a sorry excuse for staying connected with them. Think you're the only one who needs this call? Wrong! Your friends need you as much as you need them.

82

Try a new restaurant

Going to a restaurant is one of my keenest pleasures. Meeting some place with old and new friends, ordering wine, eating food, surrounded by strangers, I think is the core of what it means to live a civilized life.
—Adam Gopnik

It's always good for our brain to get outside of our normal ruts; the grooves we carve into our daily routines that are well worn and comfortable. One easy way to expand our world and our horizons is simply to try a new restaurant.

Maybe for some people that is a new cuisine they've never tried like Ethiopian (a favorite of mine) or Thai. Maybe it is trying something new in your town that just opened–something exciting and creative. Maybe it is treating yourself to a multicourse meal that is meant to be savored and delving into the layers of flavor slowly and intentionally. Maybe it is taking friends to a Tapas restaurant where the small plates are meant to be shared at the table.

Just take that small step of going somewhere new and your brain will be treated to lots of sensations and the ripple effect is that you are reminded you aren't stuck. You can do new things, forge new pathways.

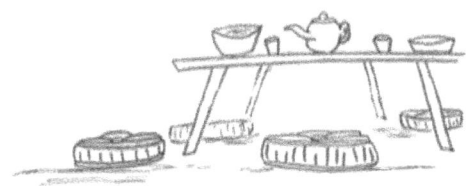

83

Wake up well

In the morning a man walks with his whole body; in the evening, only with his legs.
—*Ralph Waldo Emerson*

Nearly every self help book I've ever gotten my hands on has this in common: strongly suggesting a morning routine. I cannot tell you how many "sure fire morning routines to achieve all my goals" I've done for three mornings—only to abandon it for something new. . .or my favorite thing—sleeping until right before I have to go somewhere.

I am admittedly not a morning person. I find my creativity a little better in the evenings when my kids are in bed and it's quiet. I have come to settle into the fact that I probably will never be a kick-ass morning glory ready to seize the day, despite my best efforts.

But sometimes I need a reset, I need to wake up well, make things happen, and feel better. Those are the mornings that I will create a little 3-step morning routine for myself and stick to it for a week. It's just a week, and it's just three things (and those things can change based on what I want to accomplish). Something about the open ended nature of it, and the fact that I'm not locked in, helps me be productive with it.

Sometimes I'm trying to finish a book so I have to add more writing time into my day; sometimes I'm trying to drink water before coffee, and then there was that month that I had to dance first thing or I wouldn't get out of bed.

Maybe you are a morning person and trying something for a week might change your life. Maybe you'll do that for the next 40 years. Maybe you're like me and just need a little anchor in this wild and crazy life. Either way, mornings are an opportunity to view your day differently, to discover the magic of productive mornings or mornings where you just simply take extra sweet care of yourself. Waking up well is the gift you didn't know you were capable of giving yourself.

And guess what, coffee can be one of your 3 things. So you've only got 2 to come up with.

84

Tend to a plant

Like people, plants respond to extra attention.
—*H. Peter Loewer*

Houseplants are some sort of magic. I love walking into the homes of friends who have green thumbs and whose homes are full of sun and greenery. It just feels good to be surrounded with growing things like that, almost as if we were created to be surrounded by living, breathing plants!

I am not an expert at tending plants and yet I love trying. When I was very depressed I had people bring me flowers sometimes, which was lovely. . .until they died and I was constantly reminded of the fact that I needed to dispose of the rotting stems. Once a friend brought me a pythos plant (which are the easiest to keep alive) and I absolutely loved it. I loved how it looked—bringing nature into my home. I loved watching it grow. I even loved the tiny acts of caring for it with the random cups of water I would pour on it. A houseplant is a mirror of ourselves. The more we nourish it, the more it grows. There is even scientific evidence that playing music to a plant will make it grow more.

Get yourself a plant, with the agreement that it can always be replaced if it doesn't make it. Enjoy it, learn from it, and watch it grow.

85

Tap into a higher power

You get to a place where you begin to be guided by something greater than yourself. You stop fighting and striving (indeed the need to expend this type of energy is often a strong indicator that you are not in flow and where you are meant to be) and instead, surrender to your higher purpose and be guided from there, allowing things to happen, trusting in source, focusing on your why and letting go of the how.
—Wayne W. Dyer

Religion is complex and messy. In my own history it actually holds a lot of pain. When I took my first break from going to church because I was angry and hurt after my divorce, I expected to completely shut out God. Instead I found myself in a quiet, beautiful place where I felt the presence of a higher power that

I call The Creator in the most palatable way. I felt this higher power in nature way more than I had ever felt in a church building. I also found myself able to connect with all kinds of people who have different beliefs but who do consider that there is SOMETHING greater than themselves. It's been beautiful. I now view The Creator as the source of goodness and creativity, I view the earth as a love letter from them. I am now back at church and feel comfortable talking about God in a way that used to make me cringe. Because God is no longer something OTHER, God is connected to me.

Accepting there might be a higher power does not mean you know everything, in fact I think it means that you accept the *mystery* of something greater than yourself, which can lead to a lot of freedom and love.

What if?

86

Make a tablescape

When a guest sits down there should be something beautiful and inspiring to look at.
—Annie Falk

Making a table pretty feels like something our grandparents did way back when—back when place settings were complicated and special dishes were used. It feels like it was the work of overlooked housewives in the 1950s and yet I still find making a table pretty is deeply satisfying. And something a lot of people miss out on.

I've always helped make the table pretty for Thanksgiving, ever since I was a little girl. Not only did we use our best everything, I would gather colorful leaves to scatter on the table cloth that we would pull out of the trunk in my mother's room where it sat for most of the year. We would make place cards by carefully writing each guest's name on a cut out piece of construction paper. We would light long, tapered, white candles to cast a glow over everything.

The happiness I experienced in looking at the table when we were done was exponentially bigger than the effort it took.

So when I'm feeling blah, unmotivated or down, I will make a tablescape just like I did when I was a child. It takes minutes and it makes that meal feel important and magical.

Maybe you want to go big and host a dinner party with your table ornately set, maybe you want to make a Tuesday taco night a little extra. Don't be afraid to gather elements from outside to spruce it up. You don't need to buy stuff for it to be special.

100 drops of water

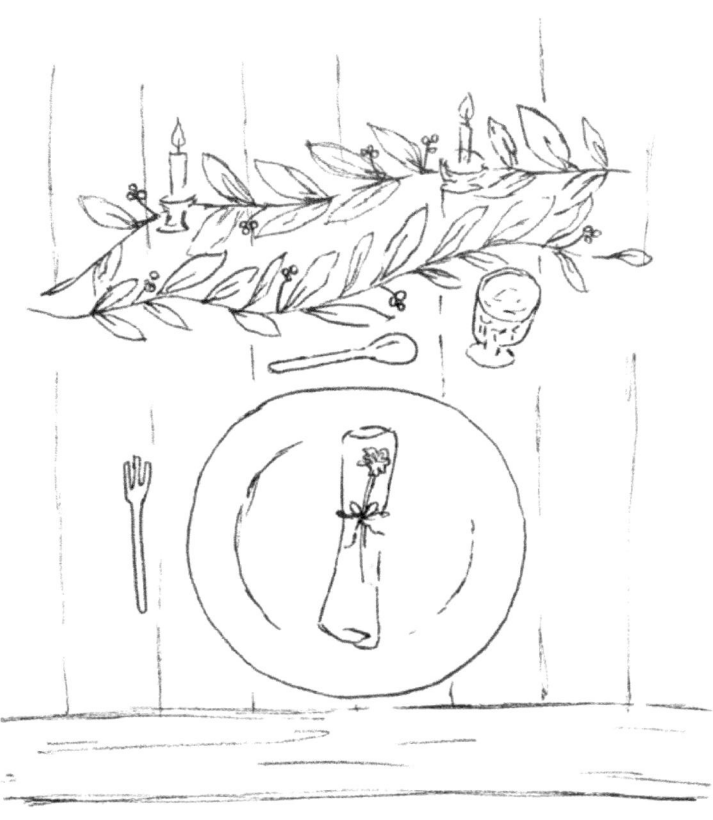

87

Make a playlist

A good mixtape didn't just gather together a bunch of love songs, but instead created an emotional narrative specific to your affection. The stories in most of my favorite collections are collected more like songs on a mixtape than, say, collected like spare change. By which I mean they are in conversation with each other and work to become larger than their parts.
—Anthony Marra

I have friends who create playlists for every imaginable activity one could think of. They make it look easy. *Drinking coffee playlist. Brushing my teeth playlist. Eating breakfast playlist. Bored on a Monday at work playlist.*

Creating a playlist can be an amazing tool to process where you are in life, to reach yourself, to make something you can enjoy over and over again. It could inject joy into your day, or give you space to grieve, it could simply make you want to get out of bed, or just to move. It reminds me of the delightful days when I would burn CDs to include all my favorite songs.

Make a playlist for now. Decide on a specific niche and search for songs that touch you right where you are.

Come up with a magical title

- *That time I cried when the leaves changed*
- *Get up, you've got magic to share*
- *Fuck this shit, I just want to dance*
- *Don't forget your childhood self*
- *The playlist for the time I felt lost, but wasn't*

88

Go to a coffee shop

The coffeehouse is good for genius.
—*Eric Weiner*

When I feel deeply alone but too tired to seek out a friend, I go to a coffee shop, order a drink and sit and observe. I put away my phone and keep my eyes engaged with those around me. I witness friends laughing and it makes me smile. I eavesdrop on an interesting conversation behind me, I watch how the barista greets regulars, I always find another person who I know is also lonely—we exchange a knowing smile and let it linger. It doesn't take long for me to remember I'm part of a whole world, I belong. Sometimes a new friend joins me for a few minutes of chatting, sometimes I run into an old friend, sometimes I leave feeling that it was enough just to be in the mix of it all.

Next time you have a craving for community, don't just wait for it, go to a coffee shop. For the cost of a tea, you can ease back into the world from wherever you've been hiding.

89

Write down what inspires you

In quoting others, we cite ourselves.
—Julio Cortazar

I was really socially awkward in high school. I was sensitive, deep feeling, and I didn't feel like anyone understood me. At my very first job I would sit alone during my lunch break and copy quotes from a book into a journal. I loved connecting to the words, saying "that's just it!" I loved the human-ness of them. I didn't feel alone when I read other people's words describing this life.

In my experience, one of the greatest gifts in life is someone arranging words just so, so we feel seen. Keep your chocolate and flowers, give me a juicy quote that fits that hole in my heart; give me the words to describe the ache I feel; give me a paragraph that inspires something deep inside.

There's so many ways to find quotes. Pinterest, Goodreads, reading full works of writers you love (I love underlining in books like a bad girl). Collect them, rewrite them, let them soak into your marrow. I type my favorites on an old typewriter and tape them to my walls or give them to friends.

Because we are not alone and there are so many beautiful words to let us know that.

90

Make a meal with what you have

The art of cuisine is the art of making the best of what you have.
—Paul Bocuse

I have this large blue and white platter that I'm sure brings my children a lot of joy when I bring it out. This means that dinner is going to be a "throw it all together" type of deal. I realized early on in my motherhood that this kind of dinner is actually not a failure at all, but something to look forward to.

I put little bits of whatever I have on a fancy plate and that's all there is to it. Maybe it's the three pickles at the bottom of the jar, 2 chicken wings, 2 apples cut up, hummus, a hot dog or two, 3 dipping sauces, and the leftover noodles from the night before.

Piled on the plate it becomes a choose your own adventure charcuterie board.

Sometimes I make soup with whatever I can find, enjoying how it feels to be creative with the things that need to get used. Or, I invent a new kind of sandwich because I have to get creative if I haven't been shopping lately.

Make a meal with what you have. This is a time to be creative and to think outside of the box. Serve it on your fine china and enjoy.

Wear comfy pajamas

I think clothes should make you feel safe. I like clothes you want to go to sleep in. I sometimes stand in front of a mirror and change a million times because I know I really want to wear my nightgown.
— *Gilda Radner*

Just because no one sees what you wear at home doesn't mean it doesn't matter. Yes I have my work out clothes that I wear when I need to get sweaty and dirty. But I also have my lounge clothes that I wear when I want to be extra cozy at home. I didn't think it mattered that much until I got my first full length LL Bean flannel nightgown. Now it is a staple in my home and it is my reward for getting to the end of the day.

Honestly, it reminds me of a super hero cape, it changes not only my mood but my personality. I also have a silk robe I don when I am feeling extra sensual and romantic. Not even with a partner but with myself. If I want to treat myself to a bubble bath with a candle and a cup of my favorite tea, I will slip into my silk robe and continue the evening. Next thing I know I'm sitting on the porch reading the poetry book that has been on my shelf begging to be read for the past 4 years.

Buy yourself a new pajama set. Get something soft and breathable. Or go for cozy flannel like me or silky romance. Mark rest and relaxation as a celebration and a reason to feel good in what you wear.

92

Listen to live music

Music gives a soul to the universe, wings to the mind, flight to the imagination and life to everything.
   —*Plato*

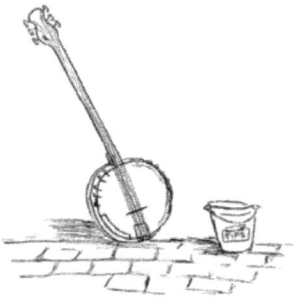

We can hear any song at any time. It's a wonderful perk of living in this age of streaming services. However nothing is quite like live music to cheer me up.

Nothing gets my heart racing like the tuning phase of an orchestra concert, nothing gets me dancing with abandon like a Celtic fiddle starting an Irish jig, nothing makes me close my eyes and reach my hands to the sky like the familiar sound of a song I love—only I can FEEL the base and feel the energy of the crowd around me.

Live music is a gift.

Some people might not think it is an accessible gift since concerts are sometimes hundreds of dollars. But there are many ways to see live music for little or no money. There are a lot of musicians who just want to share their gifts with you! Festivals, open mic nights, little breweries or wineries, local high schools for orchestra or band music, a new artist who is just starting out.

Just show up. Let the music bathe you. Close your eyes, sway, connect to the lyrics and let it spark the life in you.

93

Take a class in something new

Unless you try to do something beyond what you have already mastered, you will never grow.
—*Ralph Waldo Emerson*

There is a whole world out there of classes: painting classes, self-defense, pottery, theatre, comedy, cooking, beer making, writing…you name it, there is probably a class for it. These classes are not full of experts, wealthy people, or even bored people. These classes are full of vibrant humans who want to know more about something new, who have a craving for trying they have never tried. That in itself is wonderful…to be in a room of people with that kind of energy.

And it doesn't always end up being something that you will do forever. I took a pottery class one time and expected to kill it. I'm an artsy woman and I did assume a pottery wheel would one day make it to my home. That class did not go as planned. I didn't have the patience or the detail orientation to really go that far, but the feeling of the mud in my hands, the laughter as I failed over and over, the joy of seeing a friend doing it well. It made for a very pleasant evening.

Then I think about my friend, Julie, who worked so hard her whole life and knew the second she was retired that she would learn to paint. I was obsessed with her joy as she achieved her goal by going to a weekly painting class. She looked forward to every class and got better and better and better.

Try something new! Maybe it's one class, maybe it's a six week series. Maybe it's in person, on zoom, or at your local bingo hall. Show up, be an eager student and don't take it too seriously!

Photograph something beautiful

The earth is art, the photographer is only a witness.
—Yann Arthus-Bertrand

Stand near anything beautiful and then turn around and you will see people with their phones out or a camera taking photos of it. Maybe it's a landmark in a city, the Grand Canyon, or a radiant sun set. Photographing something isn't really about having that photo or printing that photo but it's about the ritual of capturing something beautiful.

Photography is art, it's creativity, it's painting without the mess!

While photographing big beautiful things is fun, something really enjoyable is challenging yourself to photograph beauty in the ordinary. Challenge yourself to capture 10 photos in a particular place. Maybe you'll capture the light coming through the window, your cat curled in a ball in the worn part of your sofa, the little yellow flower peeking through the crack in your sidewalk. The act of noticing and preserving it is an act in gratitude.

Here's some prompts to get your started (feel free to use a phone if you don't have a camera):

- photograph something 5 different ways (partial, close up, from a different angle, full, and with another object or person)
- photograph 10 things in your home that bring you joy
- photograph someone you love
- go on a nature walk and photograph 10 plants you've never seen
- photograph 10 details on buildings in the city

How do you feel after you have done it? Meditative? Proud? Inspired to do more?

95

Breathe

Breathe deeply, until sweet air extinguishes the burn of fear in your lungs and every breath is a beautiful refusal to become anything less than infinite.
—D. Antoinette Foy

If I had a dollar for every time someone has told me "just take a deep breath" in a time of crisis I would have 500 dollars. The annoying thing is they are right. Taking deep breaths is one of the best ways to get my nervous system regulated again.

Deepening your breathing is always helpful. It is proven to lower blood pressure and heart rate immediately. There are practices with all different kinds of breaths that we can work on to give ourselves tools for dealing with times that call for more intentional breathing. Being walked through breathing feels silly, but yet the focus it takes to breathe intentionally is healing in a way medicine can't quite reach.

Here's a list of different breaths to try (you can find dozens of tutorials on Youtube):

- Square breathing
- Bee breath
- Yoga breathing/Ujjayi/ Ocean's breath
- Nostril breathing
- Ladder breathing
- Lions breath

The cool thing about breath work (and it is work) is that it gives us a powerful tool WITHIN our own bodies to heal and bring vitality back to us.

96

Burn something

What is to give light must endure burning.
—*Victor Frankl*

Some things need to be burned. Some things need to have ashes that we can scatter to the wind and let go of.

You probably know exactly what needs burning right now as you read this. Maybe it's old love letters that keep you sad, a dress that is 4 sizes too small that makes you think of when you were thin (even though you're happier now). Maybe you need to write a letter to someone who hurt you who isn't able to read it. Maybe it's a dream etched onto paper that no longer serves you.

Ritual burning isn't really part of our culture anymore but it is so powerful.

The day I got divorced I hiked up a mountain with a jar of some of my burned loved letters. I had spent the night before reading them and then setting them one by one into the flames. It was a powerful act that took a night that could have felt SO heavy and it gave me a way to physically interact with my grief…and my relief. At the top of the mountain I spread the ashes of that marriage and watched it fly away in the wind.

What do you need to burn?

Free writing

Fill your paper with the breathings of your heart.
 —*William Wordsworth*

100 drops of water

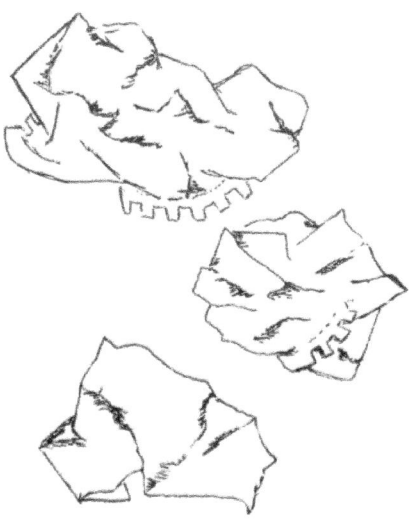

There is a method of writing that is generally used as a healing practice. It doesn't come naturally to me, a careful crafter of words and a writer, but the few times I have kept to this practice, it has more than served its purpose.

Free writing is the act of filling 3 journal pages a day with free flowing writing that you will never see or show to anyone; a completely anonymous dump of thoughts and feelings that don't have to be organized just so.

This goes against everything we are taught, that value is in it being well written, or that someone should want to read it. Much like making art just for the action of it. Free writing and the literal work of it is very helpful.

Here's how to free write:

- get an old journal or notebook (it doesn't have to be pretty)
- write 3 pages a day
- burn it whenever you want

98

Have a picnic

A picnic may well be a metaphor for life. The essentials for happiness are the right company, moderate if sanguine expectations and a reasonable standard of physical sustenance and comfort, the whole being bedeviled by the belief that there is always something better to be had if only one presses on.
—*P.D. James*

In the treasure trove of my memories, I have one especially tender one that always brings a smile to my face. I was an exhausted mother with three little ones at the end of a day that felt eternal. It was nearly spring and the weather was teasing me with how warm it was. I wanted to get out of the house but it was almost dinner time and I didn't want to cook what I had planned on that morning. Instead, with wandering in my heart, I loaded the kids up with a blanket and started driving to the national forest nearby. I went through the Taco Bell drive through and got a bag of food to take with us. We sat on that blanket surrounded by roots and butterflies and laughed and laughed and laughed.

Picnics are the centerpiece of ROM COM culture. And honestly, for good reason. Because of the romanticism of picnics with the perfect basket and the perfect food, a lot of people don't realize that anyone can have a picnic ANY old time. Eat a cheese stick on your front step. Picnic! Share an Uncrustable with your neighbor. Picnic! You don't need to plan or do anything fancy, you simply just need to take your meal outside.

Picnics are also not exclusive to couples or families with well behaved children. You can surprise a friend with one, or take your feral offspring to a place where they can run wild while YOU enjoy a picnic.

Maybe you want to carefully curate a picnic of your dreams. There is beauty and fun in that. Maybe you want to grab a sub and sit on the one patch of green grass outside of your office.

Maybe you want to plan an elaborate outdoor dinner with candles and mismatched china.

Eat outside, dear one. I promise it will elevate even the most boring of days, and make the most bland of meals. . .memorable.

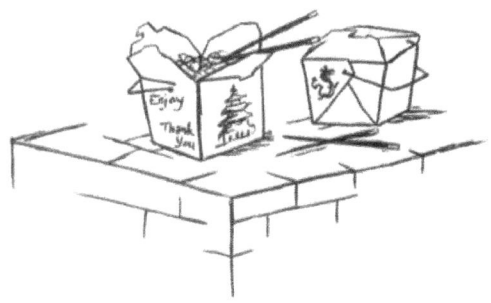

99

Give a gift

We make a living by what we get, but we make a life by what we give.
　—*Winston Churchill*

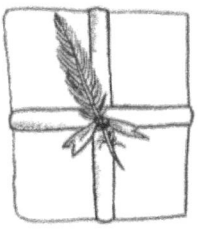

While birthday, anniversary, Valentine's, or Christmas gifts are great...giving gifts just because is my favorite. It's not about money, it's about *seeing* people, it's about saying, "I noticed this about you and I care."

Gifts can be things of value but they can also be something as simple as a heart shaped rock, or a bird feather.

Gift giving gets us outside of ourselves, outside of our small world and moves our stuck energy outward.

Since I love thrift shopping, I keep my eyes out for things that remind me of people I love. Because thrifting is random, so are my little tokens of love that I will gift to people on random Tuesdays: a shirt that would suit someone just so, a tablecloth that reminded me of their romantic love of birds, a pair of earrings, a spoon to stir their coffee in the morning.

Give a gift. Start small. Start random. Do not go looking or spending lots of money on it. It's about saying, "You're thought of" and nothing else.

Gift wrapping can be a fun little add on to make it just the tiniest bit more special. Sometimes I wrap in old brown paper or a pretty handkerchief. Sometimes I tie a leaf into the bow or splatter paint the paper.

GIVE A GIFT

You will feel good after giving. You will want more of that feeling.

100

Share your story

There is no greater agony than bearing an untold story inside you.
—*Maya Angelou*

In 2019 I published my very first book, *Yellow Tulips*, about my battle with Bipolar Disorder. Writing this book was survival for me because keeping my story inside and hidden was killing me slowly. Every word I wrote healed a part of me. It gave me the power back and gave me the opportunity to connect with other people in a deep and meaningful way. Me being brave enough to tell that story still gives me gifts. My story isn't in vain. It is helping others and is reminding me constantly that I am not alone.

Publishing a book may feel daunting, it might

make you break out in hives just thinking about other people reading such personal things about you. But there are lots of ways to share. Maybe you write it out and tuck it away. Maybe you share it with a few close friends. Maybe you post in a Facebook group or chat group full of people who will get it. Maybe you do a magazine article, blog or podcast. Maybe you tell someone at the grocery store a little bit while you wait to check out.

Just know this, there are people who need to hear your story. There are people who would be transformed to know how you got through. There are people right now who feel so alone they might not even want to be here anymore. Even if your story doesn't have a happy ending, even if you're still living it, getting it out of your body and into the world is transformative.

Be brave, start small, do not diminish what you have to say.

100 drops of water

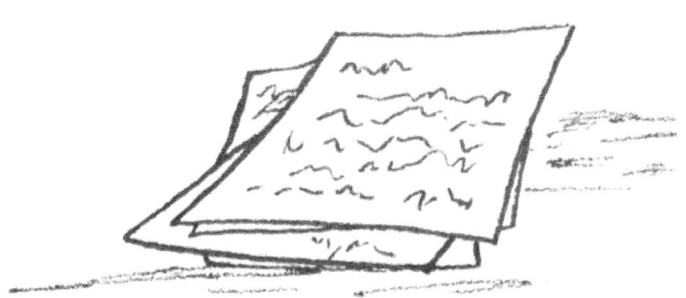

Acknowledgments

Jimmy, the ultimate waterer of my soul. Having you on my side through all the seasons is the greatest comfort.

My children, even though I wish I could start over with the wisdom I have gathered, I still treasure being your mama right here, right now.

Whitney for taking my heart and etching out drawings that match.

Rebekah, for listening to my stories and always pointing to my resilience.

Catherine, Beth, Mel, and Katie for holding me always.

Virginia, the paver of all things meaningful, who reminds me that the smallest gesture can feel like the most love.

Hannah, for being the curator of a beautiful life, even though I know you *know*.

Tori for the hugs at dance and for always meeting me where I am.

Vesna for trusting me, guiding me, and empowering me.

Melissa for always being a compassionate place for me to land.

Flo for making my books better with your editing. Your joy over my writing is such a delight.

For my dad, who always lets me know I am loved.

For Ashlyn, for giving me all the inspiration to keep on romanticizing life.

For Shawna, Ash, Kathleen, Callan, and Emmi for teaching me how powerful it is to move my embodied body.

For Taylor, Ellie, Naomi, and Steve you make my community sparkle and my life so enriched.

Also by Helen Joy George

Yellow Tulips | An intimate peek inside the mind of someone with Bipolar Disorder

Good Girl | Letters to an evangelical people pleaser

The Unraveling | Musings About Codependency, Deconstruction, Divorce, Hope, and Rebirth

If I Could Go Back | 20 things I wish I knew before becoming a parent

Follow Helen Joy on Instagram: @helenjoygeorge

Read her unhinged Substack: @notesfromanemptybathtub

www.ingramcontent.com/pod-product-compliance
Lightning Source LLC
Chambersburg PA
CBHW020534030426
42337CB00013B/851